M000014145

NO MILK TODAY

HOW TO LIVE WITH LACTOSE INTOLERANCE

STEVE CARPER

FOREWORD BY
TARUN KOTHARI, M.D.
RAVENDRA N. SHARMA, M.D.
KRISNAN D. THANIK, M.D.

A FIRESIDE BOOK
PUBLISHED BY SIMON & SCHUSTER, INC.
New York

FOR LINDA
BEST FRIEND, BEST EDITOR

CONTENTS

ACKNOWLEDGMENTS

Since this book is the first of its kind, few written resources were available to me. In their place, I was able to draw upon the expertise of many kind people in all the myriad fields that lactose intolerance touches. To all those people who were willing to give their time to help make this book as complete and accurate as possible, to my fellow sufferers and to parents of lactose-intolerant children who shared their experiences, and to my friends who volunteered to do legwork in far-flung locales across the United States, I give many thanks, and apologies to anyone whom I may inadvertently have neglected to list.

Linda R. Anzelmo, United States Department of Agriculture, Agricultural Research Service; Baskin-Robbins Ice Cream; Dr. Jeffrey Brown; Dr. Marilyn Brown, Department of Pediatrics, University of Rochester School of Medicine and Dentistry, Strong Memorial Hospital; Evelyn Catli, Chief Clinical Dietician, Rochester General Hospital; Dr. Warren Clark, American Whey Institute; Domino's Pizza Inc., Catherine Erhard; Dee Fensterer, President, Generic Pharmaceutical Industry Association; Martin Hassner, American Digestive Disease Society; John E. James, Wyeth Laboratories; Fran Kassay, Home Economist, Rich Products Corp.; John Kessel; Alan Kleigerman, President, Lactaid, Inc.; Mary Krier, *Dairy Record*; Dr. Manfred Kroger, Professor of Food Science, The Pennsylvania State University; Mary Anne Krupski, Kremens-Urban Corp.; Janet L. Lindholm, Mead Johnson & Company; McDonald's Corporation; Lois M. Meyer, Consumer Affairs Officer, Food and Drug Administration; Russell Miller, Food and Drug Administration; The Edward G. Miner Medical Library of the University of Rochester School of Medicine and Dentistry; National Digestive Dis-

eases Education and Information Clearinghouse; National Foundation
for Ileitis & Colitis, Inc.; George Nauyok, Ross Laboratories; Orange
Julius; Mary Pankratz; Miriam Phelan, President, Penguino's; Pizza
Hut, Inc.; Mr. Silverfarb, President, American Whipped Products; Mary
F. Simons, The Proprietary Association; Weiner Smith; Donna Taran-
tello; Dr. Charles Tracy, Pennwalt Corporation, Pharmaceutical Division; Martha M. Turkington, Lactaid, Inc.; Jeffrey C. Warren,
Pharmaceutical Manufacturers Association; Carol Whitlock, Rochester
Institute of Technology; Thomas A. Wilson, Market Administrator—
New York–New Jersey Milk Marketing Area; and the staff of the Science Division at the Central Branch of the Rochester Public Library,
who will now be less puzzled as to why I kept asking for so much and
such varied bizarre information.

FOREWORD

The inability of certain people to digest milk and milk products has been recognized for centuries, but recent advances in technology have made it evident that this nagging and embarrassing problem is more widespread than was ever before understood. Sophisticated tests developed over the past ten to fifteen years have made it possible to more certainly diagnose lactose intolerance in both children and adults. Lactose intolerance is now widely believed to be the most common cause of chronic intestinal symptoms in patients without serious physical ailments. The prompt detection of lactose intolerance is vitally important to us as gastroenterologists, as this condition can mimic many serious disorders of the digestive tract.

Our own research into the problem has led us to believe that lactose intolerance is more prevalent in American society than was previously believed. We have focused on a population thought to have a low incidence of lactose intolerance—non-Jewish Caucasians of European origin. As many as 35 percent of these patients, seeing us because of their history of chronic intestinal symptoms, prove to have lactose intolerance. In the past, these patients would have been required to undergo a series of costly and invasive tests to solve the mystery of why they were experiencing bloating, "gas," cramping pain, and chronic diarrhea. Our results are based upon a painless, sophisticated, and reliable test—the hydrogen breath test—allowing us to make a diagnosis of lactose intolerance in over six hundred patients in the past three years, many of whom would have continued to suffer unnecessarily otherwise.

All that is necessary to eliminate the gas, pain, and other symptoms, once a diagnosis of lactose intolerance is made, is to go on a lactose-free diet. Unfortunately, we have found almost total ignorance about proper diet both in our patients and in health professionals as well. Although we have always given out brief lactose-free-diet sheets, patients still find themselves in total confusion about such basics as finding lactose-free foods and preparing lactose-free menus.

What Steve Carper is doing here is long overdue. This book, we believe, is the first of its kind to address for the layman the many unanswered questions and to tackle head-on the complicated issues of food, health, and nutrition for the lactose intolerant. Through this handy book, you journey from infancy to adulthood, exploring in understandable terms all the important medical aspects of lactose intolerance. In addition, Steve has also provided a complete diet, some useful recipes, and a guide to adapting other cookbooks, as well as treating many aspects of lactose intolerance other than just avoiding milk products.

The author, himself lactose intolerant, has spent years researching foods and the food industry to find the best solutions for himself. We think he has done a fantastic job of educating the general public via this well-written book. We have tried, in our consulting role, to ensure that the book is just as useful as an introductory guide for all health professionals who may have to deal with this common problem. We are sure this book will find its place in each and every household as a ready reference, and as a complete source of information about every aspect of *Lactose Intolerance*.

—*Tarun Kothari, M.D., F.A.C.G., F.A.C.P.*
—*Ravendra N. Sharma, M.D., F.A.C.G., M.R.C.P.*
—*Krisnan D. Thanik, M.D., F.A.C.G., F.A.C.P.*

CHAPTER ONE

YOU'RE NOT DIFFERENT, YOU'RE NORMAL

YOUR FAVORITE FOODS MAY BE MAKING YOU ILL

Milk, they say, is the world's most nearly perfect food. Nutritionists tell us that milk is the single most important food in the diet. Milk advertisers certainly agree—their slogans are everywhere: Everybody Needs Milk; Milk Has Something for Everybody.

True enough. Milk supplies about a hundred nutrients and is the prime source of important vitamins and minerals in our country's diet. Seventy-five percent of the calcium available in the food supply comes from dairy products, along with 22 percent of the protein, 35 percent of the phosphorus, 21 percent of the magnesium, 39 percent of the riboflavin, and 20 percent of the vitamin B_{12}.

Milk is versatile as well. It can be dried, condensed, powdered, served skimmed or with chocolate added. Dairy products are used in a hundred different ways in thousands of foods, from soups to nuts and in every course in between. What's more, milk tastes good.

I used to like milk in all its myriad forms. Nothing beat an ice-cold glass of milk, especially with a big pile of cookies, made, naturally, with milk and butter. I liked ice cream and sherbet, pizza smothered with cheese, creamy salad dressings, puddings and pies topped with real whipped cream. Coffee too hot? I added milk. I grilled fish in butter and slathered butter on my pancakes, which, too, were made with milk. Then there were cream-of-anything soups, breaded fried chicken (served with mashed potatoes topped with melted butter, and corn on the cob also spread with butter), thick, rich cheesecake, bagels and cream cheese. In short, I ate like everybody else—a little too much, a little too richly, but good-tasting, healthful, everyday foods found on any restaurant menu, on any shelf at the supermarket.

I also felt sick. Constantly. That part isn't nearly as much fun to remember or talk about now. After all, what's fun about gas, cramps, bloating, stomach pain, or violent diarrhea? Long uncomfortable nights were spent wishing that the gas pains would go away, long listless days passed without the energy to do much of anything at all. I remember horrifying moments searching desperately for a public rest room. In downtown Boston, I found, even the McDonald's restaurants don't have men's rooms. It was a dark and unhappy time in my life; I wasn't much fun to live with.

Like many, if not most, people, I don't like doctors. Worse, diarrhea is an embarrassing problem to talk about, even to a professional. Gossip about pain is natural; no one likes to admit to gas. Another reason I was reluctant to go to a doctor was that the problem seemed so hard to pin down. I knew it had to relate to something in my diet, but what? I could never narrow it down to any one item. If I eliminated one food, the cramps and pain would show up after eating another. Sometimes cups of coffee (with milk) aggravated my stomach, sometimes they soothed it. Occasional days would pass with no symptoms at all, and my hopes would rise that the problem, whatever it was, had gone away. But the next day, or the next night, I would lie awake again.

Finally the symptoms grew so bad that even I couldn't ignore them any longer. I went to my doctor (or rather, I found one at a clinic) and told him my symptoms. Diagnosing me was a matter of a few minutes and a few questions. His first guess was that I had lactose intolerance. To confirm the diagnosis, he took a blood sample, then asked me to drink the contents of a bottle. I stayed within a few feet of a bathroom for the next two hours, while my insides churned. Definitely, whatever was in the bottle was the cause of my problems. Another blood test put the scientific seal of approval on the test, but my reaction was all the doctor really needed.

The bottle contained a solution of lactose in water. Lactose is milk sugar, the sugar that gives milk its characteristic sweetness. Lactose can't be digested by the body—anybody's body—unless an enzyme called lactase is present in the small intestine. Over the years, my body had gradually produced less and less lactase, until its output stopped altogether. That explained why I could never pinpoint the problem myself. Every time I took in some milk, in any one of its many disguises, I was of course ingesting lactose as well. Sometimes, if I ate only a tiny quantity of lactose, my body managed to tolerate it. A large amount overwhelmed my declining lactase production, and I suffered.

Lactose intolerance is not a disease. No bacteria or virus has invaded the body; no cells are malfunctioning or running wild. All that has happened is that the body has slowed the production of one of its many enzymes: lactase. This sounds weirdly unusual. It isn't. Drs. Newcomer and McGill have said in the *New England Journal of Medicine* (Jan. 5, 1984, pp. 42–43), "The normal state of human beings is to become lactase deficient by the first or second decade of life."

Because no disease was involved, my doctor could give me no real cure. Instead, he advised me to practice preventive medicine. I was to prevent myself from ever eating any lactose. That meant, simply, that I could not eat or drink milk, in any form, as any by-product, in any food, for the rest of my life.

My life changed that September day, mostly for the better. Learning to live without milk was a long and painstaking job. I found that eliminating milk meant avoiding many of my favorite foods. Most were pretty obvious. Every once in a while, however, I would discover hidden milk in a food only by having a reaction to it. (I think I just found some in a chicken salad—but I'll never be sure).

Since I proved to be severely intolerant—much more so than most people—I had to become fanatical about every bite of food I ate. Going to the supermarket was a combination chemistry class and treasure hunt. Days when I found an odd brand of chocolate cookies without any milk were triumphs. I learned to read the list of ingredients on every package of food I picked up, no matter how farfetched it might seem to find milk there. (I also blessed the day the government decided to require food labeling.) After a while I began to recognize the dozens of varieties of terms for milk products that commercial food processors use. My especial dread was coming across whey, a valuable milk by-product, which until then was only an obscure word in the nursery rhyme to me:

Little Miss Muffet sat on a tuffet
Eating her curds and whey...

With a lot of persistence, I found that there are nondairy substitutes for almost every milk product, so that with a liquid nondairy creamer and milk-free margarine, I could do my own cooking and baking and keep eating almost all the foods I liked. (I also discovered that contrary to what almost every medical text says, it is very easy to gain weight on a milk-free diet.)

By reading labels and cookbooks, I gradually came to understand which foods were likely to have milk added and which weren't. This meant that I could eat in restaurants with the odds in my favor that I wouldn't eat anything that wasn't safe for me. (See Chapter 6 for a milk-free diet and Chapter 11 for helpful hints on eating out.) More difficult was training myself to a new health regimen to replace those important nutrients I was losing by no longer using milk (foods to eat are in Chapter 10).

I learned to place all foods into two categories: safe and unsafe. Today checking and choosing the right foods is somewhat like driving a car. They're both so automatic I no longer have to think about each step, but I can never relax my vigilance.

When I first heard I had lactose intolerance, I thought I was alone with this bizarre ailment. I found no books on the subject, no one to turn to for advice. It wasn't until I started doing the research for this book that I realized lactose intolerance is common—far more common than even doctors believe. More than half of the world's adults—that's over 2 billion people—are lactose intolerant. Worldwide, lactose intolerance is the norm. People who can drink large quantities of milk are in the minority. In fact, milk drinking is a perfect example of the effects of evolution, for the ability to continue producing lactase into adulthood is a mutation, and a recent one at that. Lactase producers are a small and cohesive group consisting largely of western and northern Europeans and their descendants, which, of course, includes most of the people in the United States.

That still leaves room for many sufferers. Estimates place 30 to 50 million people into the lactose-intolerant category in this country. True, few are affected as severely as I am, but the most conservative estimates put the number of those who cannot tolerate any amount of lactose at 1 percent of the U.S. population. That works out to be about 2,300,000 people, many of whom are not even aware of the cause of their condition.

That is a large number; 2,300,000 sufferers of almost anything else would be part of everyday awareness. For example, the Commission for the Control of Epilepsy and its Consequences also places the number of active epileptics at 1 percent of the population. They also admit that their estimate is likely to be low, that the number could easily be twice as large; no one can be certain. But, while nearly everyone has heard of epilepsy, most people are still unacquainted with lactose intolerance. There are no organizations to combat it, no research foundations looking for ways to restart lactase production. Until now, there has not even been a single book devoted to telling those sufferers how to live with their disorder. Why? It's time to take a look at the world's most ignored ailment.

THE HISTORY OF LACTOSE INTOLERANCE

Lactose intolerance made its way into medical literature only recently, and the enormous magnitude of the problem had to wait until the late 1960s to be discovered. You would have thought someone would have noticed earlier, wouldn't you? But Norman

Kretchmer, Director of the National Institute of Child Health and
Human Development of the National Institutes of Health, has
said that "this general adult deficiency in lactase has come as a
surprise to physiologists and nutritionists..." He attributes this,
in polite scientific wording, to a "kind of ethnic chauvinism,"
but a good case can be made for saying it in much stronger
language.

The very first mention of the problem by a scientist was by
Abraham Jacobi, Professor of the Diseases of Children at Co-
lumbia University, in a speech to the Children's Section of the
Thirteenth International Medical Congress in 1900. He didn't call
the disorder lactose intolerance, because the chemical composi-
tion of milk sugar wouldn't be figured out until 1927, but he was
the first to advocate not giving milk sugar to babies and to not
follow the usual practice of adding milk sugar to cow's milk to
make it as sweet as mother's milk. Even then doctors knew that
milk sugar caused diarrhea; it was used as a laxative for consti-
pated babies.

Despite this speech—and its reprinting in a medical journal
the next year—the linking of lactose and diarrhea went exactly
nowhere.

As late as 1921, John Howland, who was making his presi-
dential speech to the American Pediatric Society, would say that
while doctors had finally made the connection, it had taken many
years and that "almost all the other ingredients of milk were held
responsible before the sugar." Howland then went on to describe
the symptoms of lactose intolerance (still not named) and even
offered the suggestion that it was caused by a deficiency in the
proper enzyme, or "ferments," as they were then called. For
whatever reasons, no one followed up on Howland's insights.

The breakthrough did not come until 1959, when a British
doctor, Aaron Holzel, reported on the case of two infants from
the same family, both of whom seemed to have no natural defense
against lactose whatsoever. He and his colleagues were even able
to say, "As far as we know such a disorder has not previously
been reported." The paper caused quite a stir and, together with
a report from Italy, sent doctors and scientists scurrying to investigate.

Over the next five years, lactose intolerance was diagnosed with increasing frequency. Two different forms were found. Congenital lactose intolerance was the type present in some babies from birth. Holzel's patients had this type; cases of it are now referred to as Holzel's syndrome. Other ailments could also apparently destroy the body's ability to produce lactase. This acquired form, observed secondary to other diseases, is now called secondary lactose intolerance.

Still, after all this, lactose intolerance was thought to be a rare and unusual condition. It shocked everyone, therefore, when reports started coming out in 1965 and 1966 that 70 percent of all American blacks could not absorb lactose and neither could 6 to 12 percent of American whites. Suddenly lactose was a hot topic. Scientists roamed the world testing a multiplicity of ethnic groups—Japanese, Semites, Cypriots, other Orientals, Eskimos, East Africans—and lo and behold, a high percentage of the members of each and every one of them proved to be lactose intolerant. It may have taken seventy years, but a pattern was beginning to develop.

Dozens of studies in the 1970s put together a fairly complete understanding of the differences between lactose-tolerant and -intolerant cultures, and why those differences took so long to be revealed. Knowing this history gives you that all-important insight into whether there is something in your ancestry that predisposes you to lactose intolerance.

All animals drink their mother's milk, and lactose, or milk sugar, is found nowhere else in nature. Lactose far precedes mankind; it seems to have first appeared about 160 million years ago with the first animals. With only a few exceptions, all mammals produce lactose in their milk.

When human beings first evolved, they, too, naturally produced lactose in mother's milk. Once children were weaned from their mothers, however, they never touched milk again. The human body is a marvel of economy. Without a reason to continue producing lactase, it simply stops, some time after the age of two or three. Until recently, every human being past the age of weaning (with presumably a few oddball exceptions) was lactose intolerant.

Sometime around ten thousand years ago, humans first developed the notion of domesticating herd animals, starting with sheep. Several thousand more years were to pass before the concept entered people's minds that the animal's milk was as usable as its meat and hide. Not until 4000 to 3000 B.C., in northern Africa and southwest Asia, is there any evidence of milking. Once it was established, however, dairying spread quickly into other areas of the world that were suitable for it: sub-Saharan Africa, India, and northern and western Europe. The Indian connection is the interesting one, for present-day patterns of lactose intolerance lie along the same paths as those taken by the mysterious people who also spread the Indo-European languages that developed into English and western European tongues.

Milk is, as we keep being reminded, an excellent food, so there were good reasons for these herding populations to continue drinking milk. In addition, milk drinking evidently gave those people a selective advantage over nonmilk drinkers. Evidence suggests that the vitamin D in milk helps the body absorb calcium. Low calcium levels can lead to diseases like rickets and osteomalacia, which may cause inability to bear children in those women afflicted. In other words, milk drinkers, especially in places with cloudy, wintry climates like northern Europe, were more likely to be able to have sound, healthy babies, so more milk drinkers survived. Milk drinkers might also have survived epidemics of cholera better than those who were intolerant. (Unfortunately this beautiful theory is spoiled by the fact that Eskimos are quite lactose intolerant. All the answers are obviously not yet in.)

The ability to digest milk—lactose tolerance—is a classic example of evolution in action over a short time, at close range, and in human beings. In every population, there would be, by chance, rare individuals who would continue to produce lactase even when they were adults. Since these people were more likely to survive and bear more lactose-tolerant children, they became a larger and larger portion of the population.

When milk was not part of daily life, or where it was converted into low-lactose items such as yogurt or aged cheese, no such tolerance built up. Of course, no populations are pure and whole in these days of speedy travel and intermarriage, but the prevalences of lactose intolerance still match ancestral populations very closely, even among modern-day assimilated Americans.

You stand the best chance of being lactose tolerant if your ancestors came from Scandinavia, western Europe, the British Isles, or a few dairy herding regions in northern Africa. If your ancestors fall into any other group—southern Italians, Eastern Europeans, Jews, blacks, Asians, Hispanics, Arabs—then the odds are better than 50–50 that you are at least somewhat lactose intolerant. (I realize that this list mixes races, religions, and ethnic groups rather indiscriminately, but they represent populations that in history have shown a notable tendency to marry within the group.) No populations are 100 percent tolerant, by any means, and whatever your ancestry, it is quite possible for you to be suffering from lactose intolerance. There is good evidence that Americans of northern European ancestry are the largest consumers of Lactaid, a lactose-reduced milk.

Unfortunately, most studies of individual groups are too small and too biased by other factors to be able to provide accurate estimates of the exact percentage of lactose intolerance in any particular group. The following table summarizes the findings of a number of studies to give you an idea of where you may stand. The boundary lines between groups are somewhat fuzzy because of differing definitions, so considerable overlapping also occurs.

RACE OR ANCESTRY	PERCENTAGE THAT IS LACTOSE INTOLERANT
Northern Europeans	3–5%
Caucasians	5–15%
Hispanics	50–60%
Other Europeans	60–70%
Jews and Arabs	60–80%
All non-Caucasians	60–90%
Blacks	70–80%
Asians	70–100%
Native Americans	80–100%

LACTOSE

Milk is no more than some sugar, fats, and proteins stirred into water. The sugar found in milk—and no place else in the world—is called lactose. Human milk is the sweetest of all types of milk, containing, in good metric numbers the way scientists calculate, 7.5 grams of lactose per 100 milliliters of milk—about the same thing as saying 7.5 percent. Cow's milk only has 4.5 grams in an equal amount of milk, goat's milk even less. There's no way to get around the problem of lactose by drinking other types of milk. Every mammal, which means every animal that gives milk, has lactose in its milk, with one exception.

That exception is the group of animals called Pinnipedia: the seals, sea lions, and walruses of the Pacific basin. Their milk undoubtedly tastes strange to humans, no matter how much baby seals and walruses like it. There may not be any lactose, but Pinnipedia milk contains 35 grams of fat per 100 milliliters of milk, or nine times as much fat as cow's milk. A famous story in the lactose world tells of a baby walrus that was fed cow's milk while being shipped from Alaska down to California back in 1939, long before scientists understood about lactose intolerance. You guessed it—not having any natural defense against lactose, the poor animal had severe diarrhea the entire trip and nearly died of dehydration.

Chemically, lactose is similar to sucrose, or common table sugar, in that both are disaccharides, or composed of two joined simpler sugars. In lactose, those sugars are glucose and galactose. No one, not even children drinking their mothers' milk, can digest lactose as lactose. Instead, as I'll explain in greater detail in the next chapter, the body manufactures lactase, which splits lactose back into its parts—parts that are handleable by the body.

Nursing mothers form lactose in the first place by combining glucose and galactose as part of the milk-producing process. This may sound contradictory. Why go through the trouble to form something that can't be used from component parts that can? The answer appears to be that the signal for the production of lactose, which occurs late in pregnancy, also signals the body to start creating milk for the baby about to be born.

The Many Forms of Lactose Intolerance

No standard names for anything occur in medicine, and if you've ever tried to gather information about lactose intolerance from a medical book, you may have been disconcerted to see that lactose intolerance was nowhere to be found. Unfortunately, lactose intolerance is a catchall name for a very complicated condition. It's not the best name, but it's so common now that it probably will never be eliminated. Still, it's worth knowing some of the different problems that can be hiding behind the simple term *lactose intolerance*, especially so that you'll understand what's going on if you read anything else on the subject.

Because it's the lack of lactase that is the real problem, many scientists are striving to replace *lactose intolerance* with a more accurate term—*lactase deficiency*. Variations on this theme include *lactase enzyme deficiency* (since lactase is an enzyme) or even *hypolactasia*, as the prefix *hypo-* means "less than" or "below." Occasionally doctors will also refer to the term *lactose malabsorption*, which applies to lactose not being absorbed by the intestines for whatever reason, whether lactase deficiency or something else.

Even when people say *lactose intolerance*, they don't always realize that there are several forms of the condition.

- Primary or developmental lactose intolerance is the most common type, which occurs as part of the normal aging process.
- Secondary or acquired lactose intolerance can occur at any age, the result of a disease or drug shutting down lactase production by the body.
- Congenital lactose intolerance is the most rare, found only in a tiny minority of babies who are born totally without the ability to manufacture lactase.
- Premature or transitional lactose intolerance occurs only in premature newborn babies, who may take a few days to reach their full level of lactase production.

Rather than making matters any more complicated than they already are, I'll use only the term *lactose intolerance* in this book. It's the oldest and most easily recognized term, for one thing, and for another, most everything I talk about in this book will concern what happens once you already have some form of lactose intolerance. Living with it is the same in every case; you need to know about the same food substitutes, and you will have the same problems shopping and eating out.

I'll use the proper term for those few times it makes a difference and explain all the different forms in their place—primary in Chapter 2, secondary in Chapter 4, and congenital and premature in Chapter 9.

You're Ready to Start

Twenty-five years of constant study have made the old ignorance and confusion about lactose intolerance almost a thing of the past. Today there are a host of substitutes on the market to replace just about any food you can name or to allow you to make most of the recipes in any standard cookbook. Milk-free children's formula is readily available, as well as a host of milk-free snacks and desserts for the young chocolate addict.

Unknown and untreated, lactose intolerance can be a miserable fate. Although not in itself dangerous (except to a very young baby), the ever-present pain and discomfort may be worse than that from many more serious diseases. The long-term loss of calcium may, in rare instances, lead to very real problems.

Fortunately, a milk-free life is easy to achieve and easy to maintain. It can and should be healthful and nutritious. You don't even have to give up your favorite foods. If for some strange reason you should want to, you can even gain weight on it.

None of this can be accomplished without a painstaking investigation of your body and of the food you eat. Your body comes first, because that's the key to understanding everything you put into it. The next chapter introduces you to digestion, and where yours is going wrong.

CHAPTER TWO

DIGESTION AND OTHER MEDICAL MYSTERIES

The only people left in America with cast-iron stomachs are eleven cowboys on a ranch in northeastern Montana. The rest of us suffer, though not quietly. How can we be quiet when we have to shout over the din of the antacid commercials on the evening news? Billions of dollars are spent each year on relief from indigestion, heartburn, gas, and a unique syndrome called the blahs, not recorded in any of the medical literature. Ask any schoolchild how to spell *relief*. Those who don't spell it R-O-L-A-I-D-S simply haven't been paying attention.

The drugstore shelves don't stop there. Our eyes hurt, our feet throb, our limbs ache, and a host of remedies are necessary to cater to each ill. From head to toe, we seem to be a mess. Even those Montana cowboys probably suffer from hemorrhoids.

What went wrong? How can this mass of creaking joints and gurgling intestines be the miracle of nature it's so often trumpeted to be? If the eye is so advanced that no camera comes close and the foot is such a marvel that no machine can imitate it, why do we *hurt* all the time? If we can send a man to the moon, why can't we digest a cheeseburger?

The clue to the answer lies back in the first chapter, in the

section in which I described how the use of animal milk began
only a few thousand years ago. Several million years of evolution
produced a human marvelously adapted to a certain life-style. In
the last few thousand years, and particularly in the past few
decades, we've subjected that fine-tuned machine to a regimen
of torture it could never have expected. Feet were not meant to
be encased in shoes, especially not ones with high heels and
pointed toes. Backs were not made to bend into odd positions in
overstuffed chairs. And our intestines were never supposed to
deal with any food quite so odd and foreign as animal milk,
certainly not as adults.

The long and the short of it is that we are genetically programmed to eat what our ancestors ate. Call it the Stone Age
Diet. The Stone Age Diet barely resembles that of the average
modern American and is not even all that close to the mythical
"perfect" diet that is always being recommended by busybodies
like the people at the U.S. Department of Agriculture.

In the first place, foods that we consider normal are completely
absent in the Stone Age Diet. Sometime in your school career,
you were almost certainly made to look at a wall chart illustrating
the four basic food groups. (You remember, it was right next to
the map of the barbarian invasion of Europe and just to the left
of the periodic table.) The four groups, according to the chart,
are those foods you absolutely, positively must have each day in
order to maintain a healthy, balanced diet: meats and fish; fruits
and vegetables; breads and cereals; and milk and milk products.
Since lactose intolerance means giving up forever one of the
"basic" food groups, your second thought upon learning you're
suffering from it might well be concern for your health. (Your
first thought is undoubtedly something close to, No more cheesecake?!) The Stone Age Diet, however, cuts out *two* groups, allowing almost no bread and no milk whatsoever—not a drop of
it, at least for adults.

Far from being unhealthy, the Stone Age Diet was terrific (as
an article by Eaton and Kanner in the *New England Journal of
Medicine* [Jan. 31, 1985] points out.) It contained far more protein
and far less fat than the current American diet (because the animals eaten had one-tenth the body fat of today's tender farm

animals). Better still, it had more fiber (even without breads), less sodium, more calcium (yes, without milk), and more vitamin C. Forget those pictures you've seen of tiny, hunched-up cavemen. They were an average of six inches taller than their descendants who lived after the development of farming. For all our advances in nutrition and medicine, we (all the adults in the world today) are still not as tall on the average as our ancestors of thirty thousand years ago. And if they were anything like present-day "primitive" tribes who still follow the Stone Age Diet, they were free of coronary heart disease, hypertension, diabetes, and some types of cancer.

Sounds good, doesn't it? By the time you read this, somebody will have a number-one bestseller called The Stone Age Diet. If not, I may take a shot at it myself. The point is that if you are lactose intolerant, your body is programmed to live on the Stone Age Diet. Milk and milk products are more of a luxury than a basic. Some of you will get very sick by having them when you shouldn't, and all of you can get along very nicely without them if necessary.

Understanding why milk can make you sick means understanding how your digestive tract works. Understanding how your digestive tract works means understanding how you convert the food on your plate into essential nutrients. Those nutrients, especially the ones most important on a lactose-free diet, are the subject of the next section.

FOOD—WHY IT'S GOOD FOR YOU

All food is composed of proteins, carbohydrates, and fats, with a tiny sprinkling of vitamins and minerals thrown in for good measure. The trouble is, the body doesn't—in fact, can't—use proteins, carbohydrates, and fats. Instead, it uses their most basic units—amino acids, glucose, and fatty acids—to supply the needs of the brain, heart, lungs, blood, and all the other tissues and organs. Breaking down food into these basic units is what digestion is all about. If what you swallow can't be properly digested, it is treated as waste and is eventually expelled from the body, sometimes causing considerable distress on its way out. We'll take a look at each of the essential nutrients and how they are digested, winding up with just exactly what happens when someone who is severely lactose intolerant eats or drinks any lactose.

PROTEIN

Most of what you know as you is protein—about half of the nonwater weight in your body. Muscles, blood, hormones, genetic material, and most of the chemical regulators in the body are composed of proteins. It shouldn't be surprising, then, that meat is a good source of protein, along with eggs, fish, and cheese, although strict vegetarians can still easily manage to receive their daily protein from grains, nuts, and beans.

Milk is not an especially important source of protein because it is mostly water. However, once the water is removed, both the curds and the whey remaining (remember Little Miss Muffet) are heavy in protein. The curds provide casein, which is often added to commercially processed foods as a protein supplement and which makes so many hard cheeses, including Cheddar, Romano, and Swiss, good sources of protein. Whey produces soft cheeses, like cottage cheese, cream cheese, and ricotta. Whey and the whey proteins are also found in hundreds of commercial foods.

Proteins are broken by digestion into components called amino acids, which are then put back together (synthesized) in new ways to form the thousands of proteins necessary to run the body. Certain of these amino acids can be built from scratch in the body, but eight, called the essential amino acids, must be supplied through our daily meals. Some foods, particularly plant foods, are deficient in certain of these essential amino acids. Care is needed by strict vegetarians to achieve the proper balance of vegetable proteins so that all the essential amino acids are contained in the diet.

Modern Americans get about 12 percent of their daily calories from protein, though pregnant and nursing women and children should get even more—about 14 percent. Children need as much protein daily as adults do to meet the demands of their growing bodies. Eskimos, who live on a variation of the Stone Age Diet, get as much as 40 percent of their daily calories from high-fat animal protein, while Africans living in drought-plagued near-starvation may get only a small percentage of low-value vegetable protein. It is generally agreed, however, that 10 to 12 percent protein a day is advisable for modern Americans.

CARBOHYDRATES

With carbohydrates, we get down to serious business, because sugars are carbohydrates and lactose is a sugar. Starches are a second form of carbohydrates in our diet.

A third group, all of them indigestible by humans, is collectively known as roughage or fiber, highly thought of in all the latest diet and nutrition books. The indigestibles pass out of the body as waste material, but on the way through, they serve several important functions. They stimulate the contractions in the intestines needed to move food along, absorb water to give bulk, and may play a role in preventing cancer of the colon and other diseases.

Digestion of the other carbohydrates has just one end purpose—the release or production of a sugar called glucose. Glucose is the primary fuel of the brain and the major source of quick energy in the body. When the body is at rest, the brain uses two-thirds of all the glucose in the blood, meaning that one pound of brain tissue burns sixty-six times as much glucose as one pound of muscle tissue. Glucose is so important that if the body doesn't get an adequate supply of it from carbohydrates in the diet, it will start using stored fat (good if you are trying to lose weight on a diet) or even stored protein (bad because protein needs to be spared for other vital functions) to produce glucose.

Lactose is a sugar, but its only importance to the body is that it is half glucose and half another simple sugar, called galactose. Since galactose is quickly converted into glucose, lactose is a quick and direct means for a baby to get the glucose it so desperately needs. Children and adults have many other glucose sources, however. Sucrose, or common table sugar, is glucose plus fructose, fruit sugar. Maltose, malt sugar, is glucose plus another glucose. And starch is nothing but a whole long chain of glucose molecules.

Starches are digested more slowly and so produce a steadier

stream of glucose into the body than do sugars. For this reason, most true diet experts tell you to eat foods heavy in starches and fiber, the "complex" carbohydrates (beans, nuts, fruits and vegetables, and grains), which also contain other important nutrients. Sugar does produce energy, which is only another way of saying that it contains calories, but it has no other nutritive value. Sugar can rot your teeth, produce gas and cramps, and make you fat. Its one advantage is that it tastes great, making it all the more difficult to take it out of the diet.

Our bodies protect us for those long intervals when we're not actively eating by having not one but two different ways of storing energy. One is a carbohydrate called glycogen, which is stored in the liver, and the other is fat, which is stored everywhere. In between meals, the liver produces glucose for energy out of its glycogen supply. For the long haul, we use fats.

Some famous diets such as the Scarsdale Diet recommend a high protein–low carbohydrate regimen. These diets are not well thought of by more objective experts. If you keep your carbohydrate load to about 60 percent of your daily calories, you are doing pretty well, especially if those calories are low in sugars and higher in starches and fiber.

FATS

Sometimes you can't win. Go to all the time and trouble of picking out a beautiful-looking piece of lean meat, cut away all the excess fat you can see, and you're still eating something that is about 30 percent fat. Eat a tender, juicy slice of filet mignon and you may be eating as much as 50 percent fat. (Check the nutrition table contained in Appendix B.) Oils, by the way, like peanut or sunflower oil, are simply fats that remain liquid at room temperature. Though you don't find any food tables that show it, you as a human are also about 30 percent fat if you are mildly overweight. Even professional marathon runners have 2 or 3 percent fat left on their bodies. They could not do without it.

Fat is the way our bodies store long-term energy. Indeed, fat is a superior way of storing energy. Fats contain twice as many calories per pound as carbohydrates do and can be packed into a smaller space. The marathoner burning 800 calories an hour for a 2½ hour race receives this much energy from only ⅓ pound of fat.

The problem so many millions of Americans have with overweight is that our bodies store fat for energy needs in anticipation of emergencies that never come. This, too, dates back to the Stone Age Diet. Over the centuries, those of our ancestors who were best at storing energy for those long periods between successful hunts were the ones who survived. The diet that worked best for this was high in fat and high in protein (any excess of which is stored as fat).

Today, with three meals a day plus snacks the norm, fat in the diet is mostly unnecessary. Without constant effort—long-term aerobic exercise in particular—the fat accumulates until none of our clothes fit anymore. There is nothing mysterious about dieting: the way to lose weight is to eat a little less (but more healthily), exercise a little more, and lose the weight slowly but steadily. Easier said than done.

Fats have one other major purpose in life besides that of being an energy storehouse; certain vitamins require fats to be absorbed by the body. More on that in the next section.

VITAMINS

Vitamins were given their name by Casimir Funk, a scientist who is immortalized in this rhyme:

> *How grateful we are to Dr. Funk,*
> *Who by science, skill, and knack,*
> *Extracted the vitamins out of foods*
> *So we have to put them back.*

The healthful effects of vitamins were known long before they were named, or even thought of, from the days when British sailors were nicknamed Limeys because they drank lime juice on long sea voyages to prevent scurvy. This "antiscorbutic vitamin" is still called ascorbic acid or, more familiarly, vitamin C.

Scurvy is just one of a long line of so-called deficiency diseases, from beriberi to pellagra to rickets, now mostly unknown in the United States, that are prevented by tiny doses of vitamins. How tiny? Well, an ounce of vitamin D is a seven-thousand-year supply for the average adult.

Vitamins can work in such ridiculously tiny amounts because they act as catalysts. In other words, they help other chemical reactions work faster or more efficiently without being used up themselves.

Neither vitamin C nor the B-complex vitamins are stored well in the body, so you constantly need to replenish your supply of these through the foods you eat. Because we can't store B and C, we are also in no danger of overdosing on them: even if you try to take more than the body needs, say in the hope of warding off colds or more serious diseases, all the excess vitamin C is rapidly excreted in the urine.

Vitamins A, D, E, and K work a little differently. They are found primarily in fatty foods and require internal fat to be absorbed into the body. Since many high-fat foods are just the flesh of other animals, it should be no surprise to hear that humans can store these vitamins as well, primarily in the liver. Fish do this even better (yes, cod liver oil *is* good for you, if you happen to need vitamin A), but polar bears are the champs. Early arctic explorers are rumored to have died from overdoses of vitamin A after eating polar bear liver.

Vitamin D is of concern to us because it is the vitamin that controls the way calcium enters growing bones. Young children who don't get enough vitamin D can develop rickets, in which bones stay soft enough to cause deformities, while older adults are afflicted with osteoporosis, leaving their bones without the minerals necessary to keep them strong. Calcium supplements should ideally be taken with vitamin D.

A proper, nutritionally balanced diet along with a little sunshine should provide all the vitamins you'd ever need. The existence of fat-soluble vitamins is the best argument for occasionally eating fat in foods. A totally fat-free diet would lead to the variety of deficiency diseases that the vitamins prevent. Even with the over-abundance of fat in our diets, vitamin supplements are a necessity for most people with lactose intolerance. I'll talk about these specifically in Chapter 10.

MINERALS

Proteins, carbohydrates, fats, vitamins—all are organic pieces of your diet, since all come from other living matter. If we were to burn off all the organic matter in food, what would be left is a tiny percentage of inorganic minerals that, as the residue of a fire, we might as well call ash.

There's not much of this ash in food. Milk is 99.9 percent organic material, leaving only a tenth of a percent for ash. That little bit is the most important source of both calcium and phosphorus for bone and teeth formation that most people have, however. Because most of the mineral matter in our body is in the form of bones and teeth, we need more calcium and phosphorus than any other mineral—about a gram each day, or an ounce a month.

At least seventeen other elements are considered essential nutrients in our diet, all in far smaller quantities. Iron is probably the best known, thanks to all those commercials warning us about "iron-poor blood." Vitamin B_{12} or cyanocobalamin has a cobalt atom in its center that puts the "cobal" in the center of its name. Iodine helps prevent goiter. And so on through such rare trace elements as manganese, molybdenum, and selenium.

The more scientists learn about minerals, the more roles they discover in the body for them. Right now nobody knows why poisonous arsenic is found in tiny traces in our bodies and in the foods we eat. Even if no purpose is ever found for arsenic, though, I wouldn't worry too much about its presence. Meat contains at least ten million times as much protein as it does arsenic.

DIGESTION—WHAT SHOULD HAPPEN

Many diet books are silent about the process of digestion, with some good reason. A fantastic number of sophisticated chemical reactions and ingenious mechanical shunts and linkages occur in the thirty-foot hollow tube that is our digestive system—far too many to be looked at in any detail by authors rushing to tell you how to lose forty pounds in thirty days by eating nothing but used pencil shavings and whipped cream.

In the real world, there is more to a lactose-free diet than the mere act of avoiding milk products, and a basic understanding of what goes on inside your body after you eat can be a real help in planning your diet.

Down the Hatch

We have a hole all the way through our bodies. The "up" end is the mouth, the down side is the anus. What is in between is known as the digestive tract or the gastrointestinal system (which is why a doctor testing your insides refers to the tests as a GI series). Not only does the digestive tract have an up and down, but it is also one-way. Some serious problems can occur when the contents of the tract move the wrong way.

Digestion begins the instant food enters your mouth. Your teeth physically break down the food to a size and consistency the later parts of the digestive tract can deal with. The chemical phase of digestion also begins in the mouth. The presence (and sometimes even the thought) of food triggers the outpouring of saliva from the several pairs of salivary glands. Saliva not only softens food, making it slide through the digestive tract more easily, but also starts the digestion of starches through the enzymes it contains.

Enzymes

All food, from the most mouthwatering to the most repulsive, is made of essentially the same raw materials. Somehow, in the process of digestion, the body has to be able to tear apart a complicated food like a julienne salad or TV dinner and produce the glucose, amino acids, fatty acids, and glycogen that the body needs for energy, growth, and well-being. Enzymes are the means by which the body accomplishes this.

Enzymes are themselves proteins and so, like all proteins, are built out of chains of amino acids. You can think of amino acids as letters in an alphabet, just like the letters in English. There are twenty known amino acids, so an enormous number of protein "words" can be put together. Just as no two words in English mean exactly the same thing, each protein has its own special function controlled by the "spelling" of its amino acid chain. Enzymes, therefore, are very specific: each has the job of breaking down one particular molecule. And that molecule can be broken down only by that one type of enzyme.

Let's take, as a purely random example, a molecule of lactose. The enzyme counterpart of lactose is called lactase. When a molecule of lactase encounters a molecule of lactose, it splits the lactose into glucose and galactose, which can be more directly used by the body. If there is no lactase around, however, the lactose simply sits there unchanged. No other enzyme will work to break down the lactose.

Enzymes might be thought of as keys, each one made to fit a particular lock. A single key of the right kind can unlock hundreds of doors in a very short time and still be useful to unlock more in the future. This is just another way of saying that, like vitamins, enzymes are catalysts. They make a chemical reaction (like digestion) work more quickly without being used up in the process. Enzymes, as the commercials say, give fast, fast, fast relief by breaking down thousands of large, unwieldy molecules into their component parts in a fraction of the time it would otherwise take. One body enzyme, appropriately named catalase, can break down its target, hydrogen peroxide, at a rate of five million molecules per minute.

Without enzymes to keep the body humming along, most bodily functions stop dead. Many quick-acting poisons, including the ever-popular cyanide, do their dirty work by keeping our enzymes from working properly. Enzyme destroyers that work only on the enzymes found in bacteria that cause disease in humans are called miracle drugs rather than poisons. Sulfa, penicillin, and other antibiotics fall into this category.

Enzymes are found in great numbers all through the digestive tract (and everywhere else in the body, of course). I won't name them all, because I've mentioned the only one that is of real concern to us: lactase. Whenever I talk about the breakdown of food, however, you should remember that it is an enzyme doing the heavy work.

THE STOMACH

Swallowed food is pushed from your throat down a ten-inch-long tube called the esophagus, which opens into the stomach. When I say pushed, I mean exactly that. The esophagus is surrounded by two sets of muscles, one running along its length, the other circling the tube at intervals like rings on a finger. Both sets of muscles work together to squeeze food along its proper path to the stomach. This muscular squeezing motion, found not only in the esophagus but in every other part of the digestive tract, is called peristalsis and is extremely important both when our systems are working well and when they are not.

The poor stomach takes a lot of grief from people that it doesn't deserve. For one thing, the stomach has nothing to do with that big pot belly hanging over a pair of pants. That's just fat. The stomach itself is small, holding about a quart when full, and sits fairly high up on the left-hand side of the body. During fasting or starvation, the stomach shrinks even further.

Neither is the stomach much involved chemically in the process of digestion. True, some proteins and fats begin to break down there, but not many, and carbohydrates go through pretty much untouched. Even heartburn, which is a catchall name for a huge variety of pains, is not always something to blame on the stomach. Heartburn can occur when some food in the stomach slips the wrong way back through the connection to the esophagus. Still, the fact that many people confuse heartburn with heart pain shows how high up the body the stomach truly is.

Food dumped into the stomach from the esophagus is immediately bathed in gastric juice. Gastric juice has two major components: enzymes, which do what little chemical digestion is done in the stomach, and hydrochloric acid, which helps destroy the very structure of the food we eat. Note that since carbohydrate digestion began with saliva, all three main constituents of food have already started to break down, even before the serious processing begins.

The stomach churns food inside it much like a washing machine thrashes clothes, reducing once-mouthwatering food to a thick, somewhat liquid mass called chyme (pronounced with a k). Though normally you can't feel any of this motion, it lasts for quite a long time. An average period is three to four and a half hours, but this can vary greatly depending on the food, the person, and the circumstances of eating. Finally the chyme disappears into the small intestine, where the real digestion starts.

Though this all sounds simple, a great deal can go wrong and often does. The problem is that the stomach is a fairly tender and delicate place where a lot of very powerful chemicals are being thrown around. Too much of these chemicals will cause them to start eating away at the walls of the stomach, causing intense pain, bleeding, and other ailments. Excess acidity is no myth. Sores on the inside of the stomach (or elsewhere in the digestive tract) are called ulcers. They can be triggered by diet, stress, or a combination of these and other factors.

When the food is the right consistency, it begins to empty into the small intestine through a connection much like the one separating the esophagus from the stomach. The muscles controlling this connection open regularly about every twenty seconds, in coordination with the waves of peristalsis that move the food around inside the stomach. Further peristaltic waves are set off when the food hits the intestines. This helps explain why a meal can quickly trigger a bowel movement even though food takes so long to travel through your system. The peristaltic waves move much faster and start to push on the waste left over from an earlier meal even before you've had a chance to enjoy the one you're working on.

THE SMALL INTESTINE

The small intestine, also known as the small bowel, is called small only because it is like a pipe with a narrow opening. Otherwise much about the small intestine is quite large, including its length; it curls back and forth through the abdomen for some twenty to twenty-five feet.

The inner surface of the small intestine is covered with thousands of microscopic projections called villi, making the intestine look a bit like a piece of Velcro. Nutrients properly broken down by the process of digestion are absorbed into the body through the thousands of villi, effectively giving the small intestine a far vaster surface area even than its length would indicate. If it were somehow spread flat, the absorptive area of the small intestine would be about the size of a football field.

The small intestine is divided into three parts, each with a fine-sounding Latin name. They are the *duodenum*, the *jejunum*, and the *ileum*. The duodenum, which is the first foot or so of the small intestine, isn't so much an active piece of the digestive tract as it is a mixing bowl for powerful chemicals. Ninety percent of all ulcers occur in the duodenum, the result of the highly acid chyme from the stomach hitting a very sensitive part of the body.

These ulcers are concentrated in the first inch and a half, because at that point the body starts sending natural antacids into the duodenum. These antacids, pancreatic juice from the pancreas and bile from the liver, have another major role. They are responsible for the chemical digestion of starches, proteins, and fats.

The half-digested mass from the duodenum empties into the jejunum, and here at last the process is complete. More enzymes pour onto what is left of your food, and they break down the complex molecules into their component parts for absorption into the body.

Included in the list of enzymes found here are maltase, which breaks down maltose, or malt sugar, a by-product of carbohydrate breakdown; sucrase, which breaks down sucrose, or ordinary table sugar; and lactase, the enzyme that splits lactose into glucose and galactose.

Let's get technical for a moment and examine how lactase works. As I noted before, the basic food constituents are absorbed by the thousands of villi that are part of the inner surface of the small intestine. A single villi is called a villus, which deserves to be looked at in depth.

Through a microscope, a villus can be seen as a fingerlike outgrowth of the intestinal wall, whose center is filled with blood vessels and lymph vessels. Surrounding the vessels is a layer of so-called differentiated cells. It is here in the differentiated cells, and specifically in their very surface, called the brush border (itself composed of microvilli), that lactase is found. Scientists are unsure of exactly where and how the lactase is formed in the villus; it is a difficult spot to study.

After the lactase splits the lactose molecules, some of the glucose is used directly by the villus for its own energy needs. The remainder, and all the galactose, enters the bloodstream through the interior blood vessels and eventually goes to the liver for storage. Amino acids use a similar route, but glycerol and fatty acids, the products of fat digestion, use the lymphatic vessels to make their way through the body.

As more and more enzymes go to work on the chyme, all that should remain in the intestine are glucose and other simple sugars, amino acids, fatty acids, and glycerol, water, and indigestible waste. Through the absorptive work of the villi, however, even these disappear one by one, until in the ileum, the last remaining building blocks of food are finally completely digested. What is left—water and waste—is sent on to the large intestine.

(If you're wondering what happens to the vitamins and minerals in digestion, the answer is that they don't require any complicated process of digestion. Once they're liberated from food as the proteins, fats, and carbohydrates are digested, the vitamins and minerals, single molecules to begin with, are absorbed into the bloodstream directly.)

THE LARGE INTESTINE

Though digestion is complete, absorption goes on. Water is an important and often overlooked component of the food we eat. Most of our body tissues are water, the bloodstream and other vital bodily fluids are water based, many of the chemical reactions that keep us alive require water in which to function. As the leftovers from the small intestine pass through the large intestine (also known as the large bowel or the colon), the all-important water is absorbed by the body, leaving behind a soft but solid mass known politely as feces or stool.

The stool consists largely of indigestible roughage: cellulose and similar carbohydrates; collagen and other connective tissue from meats; and pigments from the bile that was released into the duodenum by the liver. The stool gets its characteristic dark color from these pigments.

The last four or five inches of the thirty feet in the digestive tract is the part of the large intestine known as the rectum. Wastes gather here, waiting for release through the anus. Adults and older children voluntarily control the opening and closing of the anus, using another ringlike muscle (similar to the ones at either end of the stomach) called the anal sphincter. Babies have no control over their anal sphincters, substituting a complete control over their parents instead.

Slow Food Is Better Than Fast Food

Normal doesn't mean an awful lot when dealing with human beings in their infinite variety, but food "normally" takes about ten hours to travel the full thirty feet from mouth to anus. This is about 0.0006 mile per hour, or seventy-three days per mile. Not fast. If you think of the digestive tract as being an assembly line, the reason for this snail's pace becomes clear. Each piece of the tract has "workers" who do one specific job toward the final goal of extracting every possible bit of nutrient out of the food that enters it. What comes out as waste has been picked over with the proverbial fine-tooth comb to make sure that it is all waste and nothing but. The efficiency of the digestive tract helps keep people alive even when faced with life under the most appalling conditions.

And still, more often than we would like, things go wrong. One or more of the workers fails to do its function, and pieces that should be digested slip through. Lactose intolerance is an example of this, and if you're reading this book, you probably know how bad that can be.

Now that you have an understanding of what ideally would be happening in your body, you need to understand why something else occurs.

DIGESTION—WHAT REALLY HAPPENS

THE UNTYPICAL AMERICAN

When all the possible enzymes are alive and kicking, the digestive system in the human body is a wonder. About 97 to 98 percent of the carbohydrates in the typical American diet is digested and absorbed by the typical American. And that remaining 2 to 3 percent performs a useful function of its own by promoting good bowel habits. The sheer efficiency of the process of digestion works against those of us who aren't typical and who aren't fortunate enough to have an extra enzyme being produced when we're adults.

The problem we face is that the body always thinks that life will continue the way it was programmed for. No provisions are made for the unexpected. For the majority of adults in the world, the unexpected is lactose. Adults just aren't supposed to be drinking milk. If we do something as foolish as ingesting milk or milk products, we place food in our digestive tract that stays on past the point at which it would be absorbed by a child or a typical American. In a nicer universe, the lactose would just be expelled as waste, and that would be the end of that. What really happens is much more complicated and, for many of us, much more of a literal pain.

Imagine a meal chock full of lactose, say with milk, meat sautéed in butter, cream sauces, and chocolate pie à la mode for dessert. Not the healthiest meal ever devised, but true to the way many Americans eat.

From the mouth, down the esophagus, through the stomach, and into the duodenum of the small intestine, the trip this food takes is the same for all of us, whether or not we produce the lactase enzyme. The body doesn't even think of digesting sugars until the food reaches the jejunum, the second part of the small intestine. At that point, the once delicious meal has been converted into a paste called chyme, composed of half-digested fats and proteins, along with molecules of the sugars maltose, sucrose, and lactose.

As enzymes break down the other sugars and nutrients, the lactose remains whole. Even if a person produces some lactase, as is true for the majority of lactose-intolerant individuals, the lactase can only do so much. Any excess over what the lactase can handle means that molecules of lactose remain behind in the chyme long after the other nutrients are absorbed.

Water, which manages to get involved in most of the processes in the body and so needs to be everywhere, is present not only in the chyme but also in the tissues and cells of the intestine itself. Normally the pressure exerted by the two sources of water balance each other; they are in equilibrium. But the presence of the undigested lactose disturbs this equilibrium and actually draws water out of the tissue into the intestine, adding to the amount of liquid in the chyme. In scientific terms, this increase in pressure is an increase in the osmolality of the chyme.

This increased osmolality has two results, both bad. First, it pushes the chyme through the small intestine faster than it otherwise would go (so that as a side effect, what lactase there may be has even less time than normal to act upon the lactose). Second, it overwhelms the process by which water is normally absorbed into the body through the large intestine. The overflow of water has to go somewhere. Put together, increased osmolality means explosive, watery diarrhea.

Worse yet, the lactose is still present to work its mischief. To explain what happens to it, I need to start by backing way, way off and talking about wine and beer. Wine, of course, comes from grapes and beer from hops and barley. No alcohol exists naturally within the fruit or grains, but plenty of sugar does. Tiny one-celled creatures called yeasts are able to convert the sugar into alcohol in a process called fermentation.

Now we come to bacteria. You may be surprised to learn that you have a colony of bacteria living in your large intestine. While most bacteria are harmful in one way or another, these bacteria would be hard to get along without. Among other good things, these bacteria produce several of the B vitamins. For this reason, we have to be careful what antibiotics we take, since they may kill these helpful bacteria along with the harmful ones. Like the yeast, the bacteria are capable of taking sugars and fermenting them.

With all that lactose floating around, you can guess which sugar the bacteria will pick to ferment. (Actually the bacteria manufacture their own enzyme to break the lactose down into glucose and galactose, and then ferment these simple sugars.) Trouble is, the end product of this fermentation is not something fun like alcohol but fatty acids and lactic acid (the acid corresponding to lactose), along with gases like hydrogen, carbon dioxide, and methane.

Although they aren't especially powerful, these acids can cause problems in a variety of ways. For one thing, they aren't absorbed very well in the large intestine. Since they stick around for a while, they tend to make the stool itself more acidic. And a more acid stool is always diarrhea-producing, as the acidity will interfere with the absorption of water.

As uncomfortable as the diarrhea is, perhaps the worst symptom is the endless, pervasive cramping, belching, bloating, pain, and all-around discomfort caused by the gases produced during fermentation. The gases actually leak backward into the small intestine, where even a small amount can create pain of a major proportion. When peristalsis finally pushes the gas out (as it always does, though never soon enough), the gas is particularly foul smelling, a hallmark of lactose intolerance, and one of the symptoms a doctor will look for. A monumental case of gas and diarrhea, suffered while ten minutes away from a bathroom, is perhaps as close as a male can get to the sensations of giving birth.

Only the people with the very least supply of lactase get all these symptoms so severely. Others get only some or none of them, depending upon how much lactose they take in and how much lactase they manufacture. Because milk products come in so many forms (a lot of them hidden), and symptoms can vary so much, people can live with such stomach problems for years without ever realizing that the milk sugar is the cause of all their grief. For these people, the answer only comes with a visit to a doctor. What to expect at the doctor's is the subject of the next chapter.

CHAPTER THREE

AT YOUR DOCTOR'S

WHO, ME?

Lots of reasons combine to make lactose intolerance one of America's most popular unknown disorders. The big one is that most of the fifty million people with lactose intolerance have it without ever knowing it. How can you not know? Easy.

Lactose intolerance tends to get crowded out by the dozens of other causes of stomach distress. Spicy foods, gassy foods, alcohol, sugar, stress, stomach flu, overeating, chemicals, laxatives, and a wide range of serious diseases combine to hit virtually everyone in America at least once every year. Those of us who can't have milk don't earn any immunity from these particular disorders. We can still come down with stomach problems from any and all the other reasons. Aren't we lucky? (Though we're not more susceptible to getting other complaints just because we have lactose intolerance.)

Then there's the problem of trying to connect lactose intolerance with milk. Almost half the people with this ailment are fortunate enough to have only a mild case. They can drink a glass or two of milk and not feel any symptoms. This makes it tough for them to think of milk as the cause of their problems when they overdo it and have plenty of milk along with cake and ice cream.

The fact that milk is hidden in so many other foods makes it even harder for people to realize the source of their discomfort. Adults, who tend to drink far fewer glasses of milk than do children, may think they've eliminated milk from their diet without realizing that they may be eating milk in other forms, such as cream sauces, butter on milk-containing bread, and rich desserts—at every meal. Avoiding *all* milk is hard work; nobody does so unless it is absolutely necessary.

I absolutely have to. So do many of you reading this book. Many of the rest of you should cut way back on the amount of milk and milk products you eat and drink. But how do you know? Which symptoms are those of lactose intolerance, and which are caused by other problems? There's no easy answer to that question. But there is a pattern that should make you suspect lactose intolerance.

Symptoms, Symptoms, Who's Got the Symptoms?

The First Law of Lactose Intolerance is, The more intolerant you are, the more symptoms you'll get and the worse they'll be. Diarrhea is usually the sign of someone with a severe case of intolerance. Stools are loose, extremely watery, and often explosive and foul-smelling. Diarrhea can hit several times a day. Sometimes all the solid matter is expelled but the diarrhea persists, with only a small amount of water being excreted. In between bouts of diarrhea, gas is almost constant, with internal bloating and extreme discomfort along with burping and foul-smelling flatulence. Stomach noise, cramps, pain in the back or side, nausea, fatigue, and an overall achy feeling or depression can also be felt. These symptoms will come and go, of course, depending upon how much lactose there is in the diet. However, in cases in which lactose intolerance is severe but not suspected (so milk is still a regular part of the diet), these symptoms can be almost constant and lead to a general listlessness and depression.

Those people who produce more of the lactase enzyme will

have fewer of these symptoms and not feel them as greatly. Gas and bloating around two to three hours after meals containing lactose are the most likely symptoms, with diarrhea occurring only after huge overindulgence in milk. Sometimes it's the way milk is drunk that makes the difference. Cold milk or milk taken on an empty stomach may cause bloating and cramps, while warm milk or milk with a meal would not. Other milk products, such as cheese or yogurt, may also prove easier on the stomach than ice cream.

In fact, doctors often fail to recognize lactose intolerance because they think diarrhea always accompanies the condition. Not so. Someone with a very mild case can even be suffering from constipation. Others who test out as having lactose intolerance insist that they never get any symptoms from milk but will admit to having occasional indigestion, perhaps from a particularly rich dessert. Spotting the pattern that milk is always around when symptoms occur may take a long time, especially since that same rich dessert may be causing similar symptoms from its sugar or fat content. This is what makes diagnosis tough in such cases.

Scientists may still be arguing about the exact way lactose intolerance is transmitted through families, but there is no doubt that certain groups display it to a much greater degree than others. Having a family member or close relative with lactose intolerance is a sign that you should examine yourself closely for symptoms. The same is true if you are a member of one of the high-risk groups I identified in Chapter 1. At the same time, you will want to be especially aware of any long-term diarrhea among your young children, since it may be caused by the family propensity toward lactose intolerance. You'll find more information on lactose intolerance in children in Chapter 9.

Though the degree of intolerance (that is, the amount of lactase-enzyme deficiency) is the main determinant of the symptoms a person gets, it is not the only one. Individuals' bodies vary enormously, and so they can and will react differently even if the same amount of milk is drunk and the same amount of lactase produced. Some of the other factors involved are (1) the rate at which the stomach empties; (2) the speed at which the chyme moves through the intestines; (3) how much water is pumped into the intestine as a result of the undigested lactose; (4) how much the increased water load stimulates the intestines; and (5) the overall "irritability" of the intestines.

WHAT IF IT'S ME?

The very commonness of such symptoms as diarrhea, gas, and bloating make it tough for even a doctor to determine their cause. The sad truth is that many people with lactose intolerance go to doctors and get misdiagnosed. The very unlucky ones also have duodenal ulcers. They have in the past been placed on a milk-drinking diet (thought to help quiet the pain of ulcers), a diet that produces symptoms similar to those for which they are being treated. Result: they thought they would never be cured.

It helps to give the doctor an idea of what to test for. Home testing for lactose intolerance can narrow the field, although it is no proof. The quick and dirty method is simply to drink a large quantity of milk and see what symptoms develop. The problem with this test is that it can work all too well—you may be incapacitated for a couple of days afterward. The safer method takes longer and is more difficult. Try to go off *all* milk and milk products for about two weeks to allow your system to clear. If your only problem is lactose intolerance, you should feel much better at the end of that time. (Look ahead to Chapter 5 for a listing of all the different milk products you might find in foods.)

Either way, even if you have convinced yourself that you are lactose intolerant, see a doctor and go through a complete physical exam. I can't stress too strongly that lactose intolerance can co-exist with and can mask far more serious diseases. If all that you have is lactose intolerance, fine. Going off milk will cure you, plain and simple, within a matter of weeks (assuming, of course, that you stay off milk forever after). If lactose intolerance is just part of the problem, going off milk will relieve that set of symptoms but will do absolutely nothing to cure or even to relieve whatever else you have.

DOCTORS AND THE ART OF TESTING

Even doctors don't try to pretend that all doctors are created equal. Their world is divided into generalists and specialists. When you go see your "family physician," in all likelihood you're seeing a generalist, someone who has to be prepared to see a huge variety of ailments affecting any and every part of the body. No doctor can be expected to keep up with the enormous amount of highly technical information being generated in the world of medicine, and nowadays they don't even try. Any complaint out of the ordinary, and you're sent off to see a specialist. A specialist can be defined as a doctor who sees fewer patients but charges each of them more money.

Specialists who treat problems of the stomach and intestines are called gastroenterologists. Many of them are associated with hospitals and have access to the very latest equipment and laboratories for conducting tests. Ideally they have seen a great many other patients with lactose intolerance and know exactly what symptoms to expect and what tests to run to confirm their diagnoses.

In the real world, nothing is quite so simple. I was diagnosed on the spot by a young doctor who was seeing dozens of varied patients in a large clinic. I have interviewed people who saw several gastroenterologists before being properly diagnosed. Since you can't be assured of being as lucky as I was, the best thing to do is to try to shift the odds in your favor. If you are referred to a specialist, ask your doctor if the specialist has had enough experience with lactose intolerance to be able to recognize the symptoms, conduct the best tests, and prescribe the proper diet and health care. If your doctor doesn't know or isn't sure, call the specialist. After all, even specialists have specialists. A good gastroenterologist should know about lactose intolerance, but why take chances?

Whether you go to a generalist or a specialist, the only way he or she can be sure you have lactose intolerance is to test you. Over the years, about a dozen different tests for lactose intolerance have been devised. As Dr. Douglas B. McGill of the Mayo Clinic has said, "None of the available tests is perfect, being either invasive, indirect, complicated, expensive or unphysiologic."

A perfect test, in other words, would not involve poking needles or tubes into your body, would directly measure whatever is going on, would be so simple that there would be no possibility of making a mistake in reading it, would be real cheap, and would involve the same natural processes the body uses. He could have added that it would test only what you wanted tested and nothing else, and that it would always be 100 percent accurate. Remember that many other diseases have the same symptoms as lactose intolerance, and that you could be having one or more of them simultaneously with lactose intolerance. None of the tests for lactose intolerance will reveal this. Only a doctor with a good clinical understanding of the various problems will be able to sort them out.

As Dr. McGill says, all the tests that exist fail on one or more of these counts. If we could turn bodies inside out, testing would be simple. As it is, direct tests of your insides tend to be uncomfortable and undignified. They do, however, work the best. Everything else is just an approximation.

There are two ways in which the indirect tests can go wrong. They can identify you as having lactose intolerance when you do not; this is called a false positive. They can also fail to recognize your having lactose intolerance when you really do; this, logically enough, is called a false negative. Most of the tests for lactose intolerance are pretty accurate, fortunately, so if you get to the point that you're taking any of them, you're most of the way to a diagnosis and relief from the symptoms.

Of all the different tests devised for lactose intolerance, only two are used widely enough that you're likely to run into them. One is so simple that any doctor can do it. The better one requires expensive machinery and is only done by a select group of specialists. Both of them are indirect tests. Just on the off chance that some of you will absolutely, positively need to know whether you have lactose intolerance, I want to start out by saying a few words about the best, most foolproof test of all.

THE GOLD STANDARD FOR LACTOSE INTOLERANCE

If you remember from Chapter 2, lactase is manufactured in the small intestine at the ends of extremely tiny fingerlike projections called villi. Crawling inside the body to watch the villi at work isn't very practical (*Fantastic Voyage* aside), so if doctors want to study this process directly, they must snip off a piece of the small intestine containing the villi and bring it out for analysis. Such a procedure is called a biopsy. It works so well that Dr. McGill calls it the gold standard.

Since cutting into a healthy body is frowned upon, biopsies are made with the aid of a tube inserted through the mouth and down along the digestive tract to the small intestine. Sometimes doctors monitor the progress of the tube with an x-ray device called a fluoroscope. Lactase activity varies from point to point in the small intestine, but luckily the best place to actually take the sample is at a spot named the ligature of Treitz early on in the jejunum, so the tube doesn't have to travel through you any farther than necessary. Lactase production at that point doesn't show the variances from individual to individual that occur later in the small intestine.

Two measures are taken with the sample: One is a direct measure of lactase production, and the other is a comparison of lactase to sucrase production, sucrase being the enzyme that breaks down sucrose or table sugar. Much simplified, one study showed that lactase-producing individuals produced an average of 3.6 units of lactase, while the lactose-intolerant group averaged only 0.3 unit (some produced none that could be measured). As sucrase production was the same in both groups, that meant the ratio of sucrase to lactase was at least ten times higher in the lactose-intolerant group. Obviously the higher the ratio and the lower the production of lactase, the more intolerant a person is.

Obviously, too, biopsying doesn't quite live up to the image of the perfect test. Even Dr. McGill calls it moderately unpleasant, which is doctor talk for "better you than me." The use of a fluoroscope means a small dose of radiation, something that should be avoided whenever possible. In a small proportion of patients, the tube "cannot be persuaded to leave the stomach," leaving a pleasant picture of the doctor bending over the patient, promising the tube lollypops and gumballs if only it will come out of hiding. A further complication is that a proper examination of the biopsy sample requires a biochemistry laboratory, putting the entire procedure into the realm of large hospitals.

Balancing the disadvantages is the simple fact that a good biopsy is never wrong. If it is imperative that a diagnosis be 100 percent sound, then a biopsy is the only way to go.

INDIRECT LACTOSE INTOLERANCE TESTS— GOOD AND BETTER

THE BLOOD GLUCOSE TEST

Oldest and most widely used, the blood glucose test was once so common that doctors referred to it simply as the lactose tolerance test. Many of them are switching today, and in several years, it's possible that this test will be a thing of the past. In the meantime, the test remains important just because so many doctors know about it and use it.

Glucose is the type of sugar used by the body for energy. When a person who can digest lactose drinks, say, a glass of milk, the lactose in the milk is split into its component parts, glucose and galactose. The glucose is absorbed from the small intestine into the bloodstream and distributed everywhere in the body. If a doctor tests that person's blood before and after the glass of milk, a rise in the glucose level in the blood should be seen. On the other hand, if the lactose remains unabsorbed, the blood glucose level stays unchanged. Doctors call this a flat curve. Glucose testing is very common because it diagnoses a number of problems. Virtually all labs, large and small, are equipped to handle it.

Several variations on the blood glucose test exist, but the basic procedure is the same in every one of them. You, the patient, are asked to fast the night before so that breakfast doesn't throw off the readings. The doctor starts by taking a blood sample. Some take it from a vein, others use a finger prick to get at a capillary. Capillary samples seem to give better results.

After the blood sample, you are given a "lactose load." Any method for putting a large amount of lactose into the body will work, but usually the doctor will mix a fair amount (50 grams or 2 ounces) of pure lactose in a glass of water for you to drink. Additional blood samples are taken at intervals for the next two hours. People who can produce lactase will show a sharp rise in the glucose level in the blood very quickly, half in as little as 15 minutes. If, after all the samples have been examined, there is no rise in the blood glucose, you are diagnosed as lactose intolerant.

Despite the simplicity of the method, there are loads of problems with this test. The worst problem is that it is just not very accurate, giving results both false positive and false negative. So much glucose can be used by tissue in the body before it can reach the bloodstream that blood from veins can be artificially low in glucose and so show a false positive result. Taking capillary blood mostly prevents false positives, but false negative readings have reached 25 percent in some experiments.

Many other factors in the body can affect the test. A person whose stomach empties unusually slowly will not show a quick rise in glucose and so can falsely be thought intolerant. Diabetes can produce a false negative reading. Hormonal influences may also affect glucose levels.

The blood glucose test also flunks by being invasive—nobody really likes to have a half-dozen blood samples taken if there are better methods around.

In addition, some doctors have complained that the amount of lactose used in the test is unrealistically high. Fifty grams of lactose is equivalent to the amount in a quart of milk, and some tests use 100 grams of lactose. Besides the philosophic issue of whether the test is unphysiologic, in Dr. McGill's phrase, there is the very practical issue that a highly intolerant individual will get deathly ill for about two days with such a lactose load. Though having symptoms—gas, cramps, bloating, stomach noise, and diarrhea in serious cases—reinforces a positive diagnosis (in fact, one experiment found that the presence of symptoms was a better indicator than the blood glucose test), some nonintolerant individuals will also have symptoms after a large lactose load.

A variation that is also an improvement is the capillary plasma galactose (ethanol modification) test. That mouthful is really pretty straightforward once you break it down. First, the test takes blood from a capillary instead of a vein. Second, instead of testing for glucose, the test is for galactose, which is just the other component in lactose. Normally galactose can't be tested for, because it, too, is converted to glucose in the body. Doctors have found, however, that having you drink some ethanol just before drinking the lactose load delays the conversion. From this point on, the test is the same as the blood glucose test, except that galactose is being measured instead.

Just as everyday table sugar hides under the name of sucrose, ethanol is merely the scientific name for the type of alcohol found in liquor. In fact, it is sometimes administered in this test as a gin-and-tonic. In a lactose-tolerant person, the blood level of galactose rises sharply about forty-five minutes after eating or drinking some lactose. Otherwise a doctor sees the familiar flat curve. This test is more sensitive than the blood glucose test, but it shares all the other's disadvantages plus those of using alcohol.

Any test for diagnosing lactose intolerance is better than none, and these at least are pretty good. In fact, if everything is done perfectly, these tests may be right as much as 95 percent of the time. Still, over the last few years, a far better test has been devised, one that avoids just about all the pitfalls of the blood glucose test.

THE HYDROGEN BREATH TEST

No tubes. No needles. Accurate results. It sounds like the sort of test a patient would come up with, not a doctor. Just about everything that was wrong with the blood glucose test vanishes when the hydrogen breath test is used. Only one minor flaw stands between it and perfection: you still have to drink the lactose.

Though doctors can manage to come up with a twenty-dollar name for almost everything else, their test names are usually understandable. Just as the blood glucose test measures the amont of glucose in the blood, the hydrogen breath test measures the amount of hydrogen in your breath. What makes the test useful is that normally there is no hydrogen in your breath: a lot of carbon dioxide and water vapor with some leftover oxygen, but no hydrogen.

Hydrogen has a single source in the body: That colony of bacteria living in your large intestine produces hydrogen whenever it receives a load of undigested carbohydrate. Beans are famous as gas producers because some of their carbohydrates simply can't be digested by the intestines but are easily broken down by the bacteria. Lactose, as a sugar, is a carbohydrate in good standing that is not digested by anyone lacking the lactase enzyme. When a load of lactose hits the large intestine, the bacteria go crazy, fermenting the sugar into various gases, especially including hydrogen. The hydrogen (or some 14 to 21% of it) is absorbed through the walls of the intestine into the bloodstream, which washes through the lungs and releases some of the hydrogen to be exhaled with the rest of the breath.

Right here we have another advantage of the hydrogen breath test. The blood glucose test merely reports that no glucose is being produced—a negative measure. It doesn't say why the glucose isn't there, and that can lead to many possible errors. The hydrogen breath test is a positive test. Hydrogen is produced only when unabsorbed lactose hits the large intestine (of course, care is taken to ensure that you don't eat a can of beans at the same time and mess up the results). For this reason the accuracy of the test is far higher—as close to 100 percent as can be desired. (True, you do have to have bacteria in your large intestine for this to work. A tiny percentage of people do not, and for them the test will not work.)

Besides not eating beans, you have to take a few other precautions before taking this test. Because antibiotics kill bacteria, you have to stop taking them for at least a week before the test. Again, anything that would flush the bacteria, like enemas or laxatives, is also out. Chronic diarrhea similarly will weaken the test results. (Before you say that anyone who is severely lactose intolerant obviously has chronic diarrhea, I'll tell you that real chronic diarrhea is even more devastating, if you can imagine that.) Cigarette smoke contains hydrogen, so no smoking for six to eight hours before or during the test. Foods containing bran and sleeping during the test increase breath hydrogen as well, so they are also out. Honesty is a requirement. Doctors know that a few of their patients will, no matter what is said to them, sneak out for a smoke or "forget" to mention an antibiotic they're taking or hyperventilate during the test. You hurt no one but yourself when doing this, so cut it out.

The basics of the procedure are very much like those of the blood glucose test, without needles. You start by breathing through a mask to produce a sample of exhaled breath as a reference point. This sample is injected into a hydrogen gas analyzer, a complicated and costly machine that uses a technique called gas chromatography to identify as little as one part of hydrogen in a million parts of air.

The next step requires you to drink a lactose load. The amount of lactose used varies considerably from doctor to doctor. Some will use as little as 10 grams (about ½ ounce) of lactose, others as much as 50 grams. Additional breath samples are taken at regular intervals after that, with each one measured for its hydrogen content. The larger samples of lactose produce a reaction within about thirty minutes, while the 10-gram load needs two to three hours to show up as a rise in the amount of hydrogen in the breath. How high the hydrogen goes (from a start of one, it can go to hundreds of parts per million) isn't important, as long as the rise goes over the threshold that indicates lactose intolerance, or about ten to twenty parts per million.

However, the degree of intolerance you have will certainly affect the amount of discomfort and the number of symptoms you will have during the test. Highly intolerant people will have a severe reaction, up to and including diarrhea. Those who still produce some lactase will have milder symptoms—gas or cramps or nothing at all. If you or your doctor has reason to believe that you are highly intolerant, you should ask for a smaller dose of lactose to reduce the severity of the symptoms. After all, the test works equally well either way, and there is no reason for you to make yourself sick for days unnecessarily.

Experiments have showed that the hydrogen breath test is virtually fail-safe except for those people who either have no bacteria in their colons or have the even rarer problem of bacteria in the small intestine. The latter people will show a hydrogen peak in the early samples when the lactose hits the small intestine and another when it hits the large intestine. This double peak is the only way of differentiating them from the people who have rapid transit—in which the lactose moves extra swiftly through the intestines—and who also show an early peak in the results.

The pluses of the hydrogen breath test far outweigh the little minuses. It works well, it directly tests what is happening in the body, it doesn't require anything more done to the body than exhaling, and it is sensitive enough to work with smaller amounts of lactose than other tests. If you can find a doctor who gives the test, great. Right now the sophistication of the equipment needed means that only a few specialists are able to use this test. The situation is changing as more and more doctors recognize that this is the best way to go.

OTHER TESTS FOR LACTOSE INTOLERANCE

Doctors play favorites. They prescribe certain drugs, retain special procedures, utter private reassurances that have worked for them in the past and that they feel comfortable using over and over. Neither are they any different when it comes to tests. They may feel that a test has proved itself in the past, or they may have played a role in developing it, or they just may be reluctant to have to learn something new. For whatever reasons, some few of you might run into a test for lactose intolerance that is not one of the ones I've already mentioned. Infants, especially, are likely to see additional tests. To make sure that you are prepared for them, what follows are brief descriptions of all the other lactose-intolerance tests I've been able to search out.

THE STOOL ACIDITY TEST

This one is actually fairly important because it is the only reliable way of measuring whether infants are producing lactase without subjecting them to a lactose load. The bacteria that produce hydrogen (creating gas and bloating) also manufacture chemicals called lactic acid and volatile fatty acids. An increase in acidity leads to diarrhea along with the gas and bloating. A doctor noticing these symptoms should be alert for the possibility of lactose intolerance. Measuring the acidity of the stool is a simple test that can be done right at the infant's bedside, especially since stool is something the infant is likely to have plenty of. High acidity is a warning sign but not completely conclusive. Breast-fed babies will normally show an acid stool and even excrete small amounts of lactose in the first weeks. If the test comes out positive, a lactose-free diet for the infant should be tried to see if the symptoms clear up.

URINE TESTING

A few conditions exist, especially in babies, in which undigested lactose finds its way to the urine. If the lactose concentration in an infant's intestine is high enough or, especially, if a disease weakens the membranes where the absorption takes place, some undigested lactose will be absorbed, only to eventually mix with the water being excreted in the urine. This happens in normal breast-fed babies, in babies with lactose intolerance, and in adults with diseases such as sprue, regional enteritis, or hyperthyroidism. Finding lactose in the urine, therefore, is an indication of possible lactose intolerance, but nothing more. The advantage of this method is that urine testing is a familiar technique to all doctors, and it doesn't involve any lactose loads or special equipment.

CARBON DIOXIDE RADIOISOTOPE BREATH TEST

Carbon dioxide is yet another by-product of the bacteria breaking down the undigested lactose in the large intestine. Unlike hydrogen, however, there are many other sources of carbon dioxide in the body. What the doctor has to do is somehow "tag" the carbon dioxide being released by the intestinal bacteria. Adding a tiny amount of a radioactive isotope of carbon to the lactose load that the patient drinks accomplishes this. Radioisotopes are harmless in such small doses and are essential in hundreds of different hospital tests. The amount of radioactive carbon dioxide exhaled is measured in the same fashion as the results of other breath tests.

Still, doctors have been trying to get away from using radio-isotopes whenever possible, and so they have developed a variation on this test, which mixes a nonradioactive form of carbon with the lactose. (This form is known as C^{13} and the radioactive form is C^{14}. Regular carbon is known as C^{12}.) The only problem is that C^{13} is incredibly expensive, and so the new test won't become common until the price comes down.

Both forms of the test produce results that are good, but not as good as the hydrogen breath test. One big problem is that changing the timing of when the breath samples are taken can also change the results greatly. The radioactive carbon can also be tested for in the stool, but here, too, the accuracy of the test is lower than it should be.

INTESTINAL PERFUSION

Another test that would fall into the "moderately unpleasant" category, intestinal perfusion is strictly a research technique and very unlikely to be used on you by an ordinary doctor. In it, a tube is inserted into the small intestine, through which a lactose solution is pumped or perfused. The rate of lactose absorption can be measured over any given length of intestine in a variety of ways. Don't worry about it.

RADIOGRAPHY

I include this test only to show how far testing for lactose intolerance has come since the sixties, when doctors were still groping for ways to test what was then a new and not very well understood problem.

The barium X-ray is an extremely common test used because

drinking a solution of barium sulfate makes the intestines show up on X-ray photographs. Mixing in lactose with the barium sulfate results in a special pattern on the photographs of lactose-intolerant people known as a deficiency pattern, because the barium sulfate becomes more diluted (undigested lactose, remember, draws water into the intestines).

Radiography works, sort of, as a test, but so badly that newer techniques make it only a curiosity. For one thing, the barium solution itself without the lactose can cause a deficiency pattern to appear. For another, evaluation of the X-rays is very subjective. Still other problems are the high degree of radiation exposure for such a test, the fact that any abnormalities in the intestines will make the reading meaningless, and that this test is probably the furthest of any from what really happens when you eat or drink some lactose in the diet.

SIMILAR SYMPTOMS, SIMILAR DISEASES

No matter how sure you are that you have lactose intolerance, a confirming visit to a doctor is a good idea. Symptoms in the digestive tract are maddeningly vague: diarrhea, pain, bloating, and flatulence can have a dozen different causes. Many family physicians won't take a chance on making the right diagnosis — they'll send you to a specialist. Good doctors will do more than just run a test for lactose intolerance. In the process of taking your medical history, they will also be probing to try to determine if you have a second, more serious disorder being masked by the lactose intolerance.

IRRITABLE BOWEL SYNDROME

Imagine how thrilled I was to find out that even on a totally milk-free diet, I could still suffer from almost exactly the same set of symptoms. Worse, that these symptoms belonged to a disease with no apparent cause, no test, and no cure as easy as giving up milk. Now, imagine how thrilled you're going to be when you hear that the odds are good that you have it as well.

The disease is irritable bowel syndrome, or IBS, although it

goes under a dozen different aliases, from "spastic colon" and
"common enteritis" all the way to "myxorrhea intestinalis" and
"nonspecific enterocolopathy." Between thirty and forty million
Americans (almost as many as have lactose intolerance) have
been diagnosed as suffering from it, and maybe another hundred
million have it occasionally. Dr. Thomas Almy of the Dartmouth
Medical School ranks IBS just behind the common cold as a
reason people miss work.

The range of symptoms in IBS is a familiar one. Cramps, pain,
and bloating start soon after eating, along with an urgent need
to go to the bathroom about an hour or two after meals. Six to
ten loose, diarrhetic bowel movements a day can occur, many in
the morning just after waking up. In fact, the way to tell the
difference between IBS and some of the real serious diseases I'll
be coming to in a minute is that the sufferer almost never has to
wake up in the middle of the night to go to the bathroom. Diarrhea
is a product of the daytime only. One of the more interesting side
effects of IBS is that for many people, the diarrhea alternates
with periods of constipation.

The reason for this peculiar behavior is that while IBS may
yet prove to have a physical cause, it seems now to be primarily
a stress-related disorder. Doctors have had a hard time finding
anything wrong with the intestines themselves. Most people who
suffer from IBS find that their symptoms grow worse when their
tensions become greater. The only way to alleviate the disease
is to reduce the stress in life. The problem lies in the fact that
IBS can become so severe (pain from gas and spasms in the large
intestines can be mistaken for a heart attack) that it can itself
become a major source of stress in a person's life. For some
people, the realization that they are not suffering from a serious
disease is enough to ease the symptoms. Others will need to
examine their lives closely and see what steps can be taken to
reduce stress slowly.

Lactose intolerance is known to be associated with IBS. In
fact, some doctors believe that it can even be a hidden cause of
IBS. One study examined IBS patients who were of white, non-
Jewish, northern European descent. Normally such people have

about a 5 percent rate of lactose intolerance. Instead, 45 percent were found to be lactose intolerant. For these people, a lactose-free diet actually helped ease both problems, providing "prompt and sustained relief." Findings such as these indicate not only that lactose intolerance may be far more widespread than ever thought in the past, but also that lactose-free diets may hold out hope for a cure, at least for some people, for one of the most common of all digestive ills.

ULCERATIVE COLITIS

Ulcerative colitis is sometimes confused with IBS but is far more serious. For one thing, it is a true disease, with ulcers or little sores stemming from inflammation of the large intestines. Sufferers will notice heavy diarrhea along with bleeding during bowel movements, cramps and abdominal pain, and weight loss. The diarrhea and cramps will start suddenly and be very severe. Unlike in IBS, the diarrhea in ulcerative colitis will occur during the night and wake the victim. Though the symptoms will come and go, the disease will only get worse with time. It can be treated with drugs and with surgery, and the sufferer should make every effort to do so. There is evidence to suggest that the longer one has the disease, the greater the risk of contracting cancer.

CROHN'S DISEASE

Crohn's disease can strike anywhere in the digestive tract, but most usually in the small intestine. If it does hit there, the symptoms can be almost identical to those of lactose intolerance— diarrhea (with or without blood), cramps, abdominal pain. All the layers of the intestine can become inflamed and covered with ulcers. These allow blood, protein, and fluids to leak through the inflamed layers into the intestine, leading to anemia, weight loss, and malnutrition. Surgery is called for at this point, but unfortunately, Crohn's disease can recur after surgery. This is a serious ailment, but one that is less common than ulcerative colitis. Estimates are that one adult in three thousand has Crohn's disease, while about one in a thousand has ulcerative colitis.

CANCER OF THE COLON

We have progressed from lactose intolerance through worse and worse diseases until we end at the scariest of them all. Half the people with cancer of the colon or large intestine will not live for more than five years. This is still a big improvement over the past and is due to the use of cancer-retarding drugs and chemotherapy.

Bleeding from the rectum can be caused by many things and is likely to mean nothing more than hemorrhoids. Even so, rectal bleeding or blood with the stool is one of the major warning signs of colon cancer. For adults over the age of forty, or people who have a family history of colon cancer, an annual physical exam is hardly a luxury.

A diagnosis of lactose intolerance shouldn't be made without a complete physical to rule out all the much more serious diseases whose symptoms are mimicked by lactose intolerance.

CHAPTER FOUR

SIX MORE REASONS TO STAY AWAY FROM MILK

This book is for the majority of people in the world: those who have lost the ability to digest lactose as they grew older. Practically speaking, however, the advice you'll find in this book on removing the lactose and other milk by-products from your life will work no matter what reason you have for wanting to do so. And there are terrific reasons—specifically, five other disorders that also require a lactose-free diet. Those five are secondary lactose intolerance, milk protein allergy, milk fat intolerance, glucose-galactose malabsorption, and galactosemia. I'll also talk briefly about some of the religious and personal beliefs that require an abstinence from milk products.

Another book the size of this one would be necessary to treat all these other reasons with the thoroughness with which I'm examining lactose intolerance. What I'll say here is merely an overview, enough to let you recognize yourself and your situation, or to alert you to go to a doctor if you suspect any of these problems in yourself or a member of your family. Even if you are reading this book for reasons other than lactose intolerance, all the other chapters in the book, except possibly Chapter 7, contain information you'll find very useful to know.

SECONDARY LACTOSE INTOLERANCE

Secondary lactose intolerance was known and understood long before doctors realized how many normal adults suffered from primary lactose intolerance. It's a side effect from what might be described as a serious shock to the small intestine. Lactase is manufactured right at the outermost tips of the fingerlike projections called villi that line the small intestine. This is an extremely vulnerable spot. Any outside force that might damage the lining of the intestine will probably also knock out the body's ability to produce lactase.

Causes of secondary lactose intolerance fall into three main groups: surgery, diseases, and drugs. Since secondary lactose intolerance is a complication resulting from some more serious problem, you won't necessarily have to deal with it on your own. Once the usual symptoms (gas, bloating, cramps, possible diarrhea) start, an alert doctor should immediately realize what is going wrong.

That's a big *should*, of course. If you're in bed in a hospital, if you have doctors observing you, if there is a dietician on call, then and only then will diagnosis be quick and simple. It can just as easily happen that you leave the hospital within days of a simple surgical procedure, slowly resume a normal diet, and only gradually realize that you are having symptoms you never had before. A conscientious doctor will have prepared you for the possibility of contracting secondary lactose intolerance so that you know what's happening to you. No matter. If the symptoms start, get back to your doctor and let him or her know.

For most people, the cure involves a temporary removal of lactose from the diet. Recover from the surgery, cure the disease, stop taking the drug, whatever is causing the condition, and secondary lactose intolerance soon goes away.

With a few exceptions. In acute gastroenteritis, the intolerance may linger for four months. Surgery that removes enough of the intestines to make absorption of lactose impossible (short bowel syndrome) will necessarily result in permanent lactose intoler-

ance. Alcoholism may reduce lactase production at the same time the alcoholic is directed to drink large quantities of milk to reduce the effects of alcohol-induced ulcers or gastritis, giving the alcoholic a double whammy. Long-term effects like these have to be treated the same way as any other lactose intolerance—by following a long-term lactose-free or at least lactose-reduced diet.

What follows is a listing of the various causes of secondary lactose intolerance I've been able to dig up. More are certain to be found in the future. Others, including some I've specifically listed, may someday be taken off the list. (Sorry, but there is simply no room to go into what each of these diseases—some extremely exotic—is; ask your doctor if you think any might conceivably apply to you.)

SURGERY: gastric surgery, intestinal surgery, short bowel syndrome, antrectomy with a Billroth II anastomosis

DISEASES: intestinal bacterial or viral infection, giardiasis, gluten- or protein-sensitive enteropathy, tropical sprue, celiac sprue, viral gastroenteritis, kwashiorkor, intractable diarrhea of infancy, blind loop syndrome, Crohn's disease, irritable bowel syndrome, hyperthyroidism, malnutrition or starvation

DRUGS: neomycin sulfate (brand names Mycifradin, Neobiotic), kanamycin, other broad-spectrum antibiotics, colchicine, and quinidine compounds

OTHER: enteritis caused by irradiation of the abdomen

Some supposed causes of secondary lactose intolerance that are no longer thought to be culprits include duodenal ulcer, ulcerative colitis, viral hepatitis, diabetes mellitus, and cystic fibrosis.

MILK PROTEIN ALLERGY

Sara was eight months old before she had her first taste of cow's milk. Weaning has to start sometime, though, and so Sara's mother tried her out on a small amount of 2 percent milk. Poor Sara. Within minutes, she was blown up like a balloon, her eyes swollen shut. The doctor had to give her an antihistamine.

A couple of months later, her mother tried again with cheese.

In the emergency ward, Sara was given epinephrin to control another bout of swelling. The slightest bit of milk, even in other products, would start her wheezing or cover her with giant hives.

Sara became asthmatic at eighteen months. Three months after that, she developed bronchitis. The pediatrician told Sara's mother to check in with an allergist. Sara was given a full slate of skin tests, followed by another round of tests involving interdermal (into the skin) injections. The verdict was unmistakable. Sara had high allergy potential. She reacted to oats and to artificial flavoring (and to real maple). Red food dye turned her hyperactive. And she was violently allergic to milk.

Milk protein allergy is an entirely different problem than lactose intolerance. It involves a sensitivity to the proteins found specifically in cow's milk—other milks, especially mother's milk, will be tolerated just fine. The allergic reaction will show up as soon as a person starts drinking milk. Since very few Americans manage to become adults before their first taste of milk, milk protein allergy is discovered almost exclusively among children. Somewhere between 1 percent and 3 percent—perhaps fifty thousand—of the babies born in the United States each year are so allergic. However, for whatever reasons, a few more cases are discovered in older children and even in adults.

Sara, for all her ills, is lucky. Her mother breast-fed her for eight months. Despite a modest revival in recent years, the number of women breast-feeding their babies has dropped precipitously from the days when all mothers nursed their newborns. Even those mothers who breast-feed often do not do so for very long, or at least alternate between mother's milk and formula. With more babies receiving more cow's milk at an earlier age, cow's milk allergy has been on the rise for years. And the consequences of milk allergy are worse for a very young infant than for an older one like Sara.

WHY ALLERGIES?

As noted in Chapter 2, the human body is not designed to use food whole. It has to be broken down to its most basic components first. These relatively simple molecules—amino acids, sugars, fatty acids—are the same everywhere, in all animals. More com-

plicated combinations of these molecules—proteins, for example—are individual. Humans have theirs, cows have theirs, and disease-producing bacteria have still others. If some of these proteins happen to leak into the bloodstream before being broken down into amino acids, the body doesn't bother to distinguish between the good and the bad; it simply assumes that all of them are harmful. As a result, the body manufactures antibodies that get rid of the foreign proteins.

Even after all the proteins have been destroyed, the antibodies stay in the bloodstream, just in case. Unfortunately, this means that at times the body becomes "sensitized." If even a tiny amount of that protein finds its way back into the bloodstream, the body gears up and produces massive amounts of antibodies, whether they're really needed or not. The result can be a stupendous variety of symptoms, most of them unpleasant, a few of them life threatening.

Cow's milk contains more than twenty-five different proteins that infants can become allergic to. Each can cause different problems, but it is almost impossible to determine which particular one is the cause. At best, a doctor can say that the allergy comes from one of two groups of milk proteins, those from whey or those from casein. If the group to which the child is allergic is known, then only those foods containing that protein group need to be avoided.

SYMPTOMS

Allergies are perhaps the most spectacularly individual of all ailments. They can cause virtually any kind of problem anywhere in the body. Doctors who go in for glib generalizations shouldn't become allergists. The best (also the only) full book I know of on this particular set of allergies, *Allergies to Milk* by Drs. Sami L. Bahna and Douglas C. Heiner (for doctors only—very hard going), devotes a full thirty pages to the chapter on symptoms. Only one infant is known to have suffered alopecia—complete loss of the hair on the scalp, eyebrows, and eyelashes—but some of the other forty-nine symptoms they list are a bit more common.

Vomiting, diarrhea, and stomach pain are the typical warning signs of an infant who is allergic to milk. (These symptoms are nearly identical to those of lactose intolerance. However, lactose intolerance doesn't produce the variety of other symptoms that an allergy can cause.) Over half, and perhaps as many as 90 percent, of those with milk allergy show digestive problems. Vomiting usually occurs within an hour after drinking milk and can be quite severe, leading to dehydration. Diarrhea is frequent, and the loose stools are yellow or green; they can also contain mucus or blood. Colicky babies may awaken during the night with cramps that don't go away. Even if they appear to be hungry, more milk simply causes them to start screaming again.

The next most common set of symptoms are breathing problems. Rhinitis (which is a stuffed, runny nose), a chronic cough, bronchitis, or asthma occur in about 10 to 30 percent of children with cow's milk allergy. All these symptoms tend to be long-term, and while treating the symptoms can give temporary relief, the problem can get no better as long as milk is in the diet.

Rashes and hives (or atopic dermatitis and urticaria—I had to buy a medical dictionary to get through *Allergies to Milk*) are classic allergy symptoms. You wouldn't expect milk allergy to leave them out, and you won't be disappointed. Rashes may be one of the most common symptoms of all, although they show up less frequently in children over the age of two than in those under. Hives occur much less frequently than rashes and are more likely in older children.

Other symptoms range from anemia to bed-wetting to severe shock. A few doctors have theorized that sudden infant death syndrome ("crib death," or SIDS) is caused by babies going into shock when given cow's milk shortly before sleeping. The evidence, like all evidence in the tragedy that is SIDS, is mixed, and the theory remains no more than a theory at this point.

Diagnosing Milk Allergy

There are several important differences between milk protein allergy and congenital lactose intolerance, in which babies are born without the enzyme needed to digest milk. First and foremost, milk protein allergy is far more common. Second, the very best food for a baby with milk protein allergy is milk—mother's milk. Mother's milk is high in lactose, so it is deadly for the infant with congenital lactose intolerance but perfect for the one suffering from milk allergy. (When I say milk protein allergy, I'm using shorthand for *cow's* milk protein allergy. Other kinds of milk are usually perfectly okay. Breast-feeding not only holds many psychological advantages for a baby, but it also provides the infant a better and safer food.)

Milk protein allergy is usually diagnosed by the change in a baby once breast-feeding has stopped. Doctors will take into account the symptoms, ask if there is a family history of allergies (a younger brother or sister has a one-in-three chance of having problems with cow's milk if an older child has), and run a test similar to the one used in testing for lactose intolerance—a large glass of milk and stand back.

In addition, there are also specialized allergy tests. The most common of these scratches or pricks the skin (often on the back) with a tiny amount of the substance thought to be causing the problem. The type of reaction tells much about the type of allergy. Skin tests are preceded by taking the baby off milk for four weeks (longer if only occasional symptoms had been noticed). Not only can the doctor see if there is an improvement during this period, but the test is somewhat more sensitive if the infant has not constantly been drinking milk and suffering symptoms.

The skin test is very much like the blood glucose test for lactose intolerance. They both are very common, are known to almost all doctors, and fail too high a percentage of the time. Many, many more allergy tests have been developed, with different types for different varieties of allergies. Go to a good allergist and let him or her choose the proper one.

No More Milk

Older children and adults who have milk protein allergy can follow a standard milk-free diet and need only a calcium supplement. Babies cannot. An infant young enough to need nothing but milk used to have a big problem if breast-feeding wasn't available. Today the infant (and his or her mother) has a wide variety of alternatives.

First, remove all cow's milk from the child's diet. (With one exception: people allergic only to the whey proteins may be able to tolerate boiled or evaporated milk. As one doctor said, it gives them a "whey out." Those sensitive to casein, however, should not try this.) In a few cases, in older patients, incompletely cooked beef will also cause symptoms. In a very few people, contact with live cows or cow hair products like mohair will trigger respiratory allergies.

Any number of soybean "milks" are on the market today. I'll have a lot more to say about these in Chapter 6. Most children will accept them, their nutritive value is similar to that of cow's milk, and they can even be used in baking. They do have one drawback: Since they are made of the protein in soy, some humans can and do become allergic to them. About one-fourth of milk-sensitive patients wind up allergic to soy protein after using it for a long time.

What then? Well, don't panic; there are options. Mead-Johnson's Pregestimil and Nutramigen contain digested casein, which is less allergenic than undigested protein. Synthetic amino acids (the building blocks of protein) are in Vivonex from Eaton (called an elemental diet), which even comes in an unflavored version for infants with allergies to food flavorings.

No More Milk?

Now for the good news. Infants may be more prone to milk protein allergy just because their digestive systems are not yet mature. Many studies have shown that for infants who were never breast-fed, allergy to milk lessens when the baby is a few months old. For some it is gone, or nearly so, by the time the child reaches the age of one or two. If the child can tolerate a very small amount of milk by then, milk can slowly and gradually be worked back into the diet. The odds on this are good, if not terrific. In various studies, 17 to 65 percent of allergic infants were able to tolerate one form of milk or another by the end of their first year of life. It didn't even seem to matter how severe the symptoms had been in the first place.

Here's another plug for breast-feeding. Milk allergy tends to be milder and not last as long in infants who were breast-fed or who were put on a milk-free diet at a very early age.

For the unfortunate, milk allergies will linger on. One odd point is that the child may outgrow one symptom and develop another, completely different: asthma instead of rashes, or runny nose instead of diarrhea. The number of those who remain extremely allergic to milk even as adults seems to be quite small, however.

As their sufferers know so well, allergies tend to come in clusters. Like Sara, people can be allergy prone and pick up one allergy after another until the whole world becomes a trap to be avoided. A new crop of allergies may at times be related to milk, even after milk has been put back into the diet because it no longer seems to be causing problems. Another milk-free diet can be a helpful test in controlling these new allergies.

MILK FAT INTOLERANCE

You say you've never heard of anyone being allergic to milk fat? You're in good company. The most exalted specialists in the field can't agree whether milk fat (or milk lipid) intolerance exists at all.

It does. Carper's First Law: If it exists, someone can be found to be allergic to it. (Carper's Corollary: The one product you are not allergic to will be removed from the supermarket shelves tomorrow.)

Milk fat intolerance produces the same symptoms—stomach pain and diarrhea—as lactose intolerance, and a few people almost certainly have both. A group of doctors in France decided to run a complicated series of experiments to see if they could sort the two out. (The French, say the doctors—like the Spanish and Italians—find skimmed milk more "digestible" than regular milk, which suggests that milk fat is the problem.)

Briefly, the doctors tested a group of 100 brave volunteers (most of them known to be lactose intolerant) with whole milk, low-lactose milk, low-fat milk, and milk proteins. Thirty-nine were intolerant to all four varieties of milk. Twenty-four proved to be intolerant only to lactose. And 9 of the 100 showed symptoms only when they drank milk containing milk fat. (The rest showed either no symptoms or confusing ones. It's interesting to note that 6 of those who showed no symptoms whatsoever to any kind of milk were the ones known to be lactose intolerant through the highly accurate hydrogen breath test.)

While everyone concerned could wish for a clearer set of results, there's little question that milk fat is going to cause a problem for some people. For those who are lactose intolerant, this may mean that they should give up even those products that contain milk fat but no other source of milk. Even those who are cleared by a lactose tolerance test may need to give up (or may have already given up) on whole milk if it causes diarrhea or other problems.

Without a better understanding of how milk fat intolerance is caused, what the effects are, or what the range of degree of intolerance is, little more can be said on the subject now. Fortunately, skim and low-fat milks are common products already on the market. If in doubt, try them.

GLUCOSE-GALACTOSE MALABSORPTION

The problem in lactose intolerance is that the intestines do not split the lactose into its component parts, glucose and galactose, for absorption into the body. Turn that problem around. What if the lactose split perfectly well, but the resulting glucose and galactose could not be absorbed for some reason? When precisely that condition occurs, it is known as glucose-galactose malabsorption.

The disorder is discovered in babies in the same way lactose intolerance is—by the appearance of severe diarrhea beginning shortly after birth and continuing until all milk is eliminated from the system. In some ways, it is worse than lactose intolerance, because other important carbohydrates, including table sugar and starches, also break down to glucose. All these difficult-to-avoid carbohydrates must also be kept from the diet except in the smallest amounts. Fortunately, fructose (fruit sugar) is tolerated by most, though not all, sufferers of glucose-galactose malabsorption. By the age of three to five years, the body usually learns to live with the problem, and the chronic diarrhea disappears.

Because the inability to drink any milk is potentially life threatening, this condition is usually diagnosed almost immediately in infants. A few older children and even some adults may develop it. The standard lactose-free diet will prevent recurrence of its symptoms if other carbohydrates are avoided as well. You should note that since a completely different disorder is involved, the lactase capsules that help lactose intolerant people to drink some milk are totally ineffective for those with glucose-galactose malabsorption.

GALACTOSEMIA

This disorder is similar in many ways to glucose-galactose malabsorption. Again, lactose is easily broken down to glucose and galactose. This time the enzyme that converts galactose to glucose is missing. As the galactose rapidly accumulates in the blood and body tissues, it can lead to liver damage or mental retardation. Because this is a genetic disease, doctors actively look for it even before the baby is born. Tests have also been developed to screen for it at birth by examining the blood in the umbilical cord. It is, thankfully, an extremely rare disease.

One further note: the use of lactase capsules in milk is actually dangerous for persons with this condition. A completely lactose-free diet must be followed rigorously.

AVOIDING MILK FOR RELIGIOUS AND SOCIAL REASONS

All through this book I'm assuming that you're avoiding milk because of one physical ailment or another. Many people, however, *choose* to avoid milk, and the advice I give on living a milk-free life is just as applicable to them.

Although there are undoubtedly many individualistic reasons for staying away from milk products, two large groups in our society do so out of conviction.

Orthodox Jews are bound by a commandment not to mix meat and milk at the same meal. Strict vegetarians, who do not eat any foods derived from animals, have equal incentive to search out foods that contain no milk products.

Though not every chapter in this book is as valuable to members of these groups as it would be to the lactose intolerant, the next two chapters, which list all the milk product derivatives and milk product substitutes I am aware of, provide crucial information on milk that is not available in any other one place. Chapter 10, which lists the nutrients normally gained from milk products, and alternate foods that are high in them, is also one anyone refraining from milk products should read.

CHAPTER FIVE

THE FINE PRINT ON YOUR FOOD

When you walk down the aisles at a supermarket, you have to be strong to resist the come-ons from the fabulous pictures and enticing slogans on all the packaged foods. Being lactose intolerant, however, gives you all the incentive you need to refrain from unthinkingly tossing another great-sounding food into your shopping cart. Lactose is never mentioned, never pictured on the front; the only way to know of its existence is to study that fine type on the back or sides of the package.

The government, through the Food and Drug Administration (FDA) and a couple of other agencies, requires all packaged food to include an ingredients list on every label, and here the smart shopper learns all that was left unsaid by the marketers on the front of the package. These listings aren't perfect, and a few cagey manufacturers manage to sneak around them or even flat-out lie in them, but they're lifesavers for those of us who are lactose intolerant.

TRUTH IN LABELING

Even on the front of the package, the government places a few constraints on the manufacturer that help us. The product must have a name, for one thing. While this sounds ridiculously obvious, product names actually give important clues to the true nature of what's inside.

Take pretzels for example. Pretzels are pretty much flour and water and salt, and so should make a good snack food for the lactose intolerant. They do; but why stop here? Manufacturers don't. Several of them sell butter-flavored pretzels, presumably because consumers think butter lends a better flavor. Butter is butter, but butter flavor is a slippery concept. Does it come from adding butter or from natural butter flavor or from artificial butter flavor? The government says you have to know. If the flavor is artificial, the name of the product has to say so.

The result is a product like Keebler Artificially Flavored Butter Pretzel Braids, a milk-free pretzel. True, on the front of the package the word *butter* is in large type and *artificially flavored* is in the tiny, hard-to-read type that humorist S. J. Perelman once labeled 4-point myopia; even so, the *artificial* is a dead giveaway. Butter seekers may feel cheated, but it's a zero sum world—what's bad for butter eaters is good for the lactose intolerant.

This truth-in-labeling law sometimes results in mile-long tongue-twisters such as Country Time Non-Carbonated Ready to Drink Lemonade Flavor Drink, but the idea is a sound one. A product name should be truly descriptive of what it is. Combination products must be named so that the product with the greatest weight comes first: Gravy and Sliced Beef has more gravy than beef. Terms such as *low-calorie* or *reduced calorie* can only be used on products meeting certain conditions, so that you know you really are getting fewer calories for your money. The word *imitation* must be used on foods when they are not as nutritious as the products they resemble.

Sadly, not all the terms manufacturers use have such specific meanings. Modern fad names like *natural, organic, health food*, and *lite* can be slapped on any product the manufacturer can get you to buy. "Hi-energy" foods aren't magical elixirs to pep you up; they're merely foods high in calories, since food energy *is* calories.

Playing Games with the Fine Print

The only way to really be sure of what is in the food you buy is to read the ingredients list. These lists have only been required for a relatively few years, a triumph of the consumer movement of the 1960s. Nothing—absolutely nothing—is more important than these lists to those of us with lactose intolerance. If you really want to lead a milk-free life, or even if you want to be able to cut down on milk products when you choose to, you must learn how to read these lists—and then you must read them—every time, on every package, for everything you buy. I'll be saying this a dozen times more. It's that important.

Ingredients lists can't be just random listings of whatever happens to be in the recipe. The ingredients must be listed in order by weight, with the item with the greatest weight listed first. This restriction has to make some manufacturers unhappy. Because of it, you can figure out much more about their products than they would like you to.

One brand of frosting, for example, features a "made with real butter" slogan across its front. Butter is used, but it's well down the list. Margarine, however, is second.

The laws regulating the writing of the ingredients lists provide a number of loopholes large enough to admit milk products. Some ingredients are themselves made up of other ingredients. Margarine, for example, may be made with milk products but doesn't have to be. Some semisweet chocolate morsels are similarly not milk free. When such ingredients are added to other products, manufacturers are supposed to spell out everything that they contain as well, according to the FDA. Many don't. When margarine is high on a list, it will probably have its ingredients specified, but not when it is found near the bottom. In the same way, semisweet chocolate morsels may show up on an ingredients list without you having any way to know if they are milk free or not. On a reduced-lactose diet, you might want to take the chance, because the amount of lactose is undoubtedly low either way, but if you were being very strict, you would have to pass up a product that could be perfectly safe.

Informative as they are, ingredients lists still don't tell you how much of any ingredient has been added. You can pretty well assume that in a long listing, the last few ingredients are there in relatively tiny amounts, but determining exactly how tiny is impossible. For this reason, many people prefer to avoid all products containing lactose, even if the odds are good that the lactose in any one of them is too small to be harmful.

The Dairy in "Nondairy"

So-called *nondairy* products form another trap for the lactose intolerant. Nondairy isn't a term mandated by the FDA. Instead, its use is required by certain states when milk proteins like casein or sodium caseinate are the sole milk-derived ingredients in a product that is a milk substitute. The idea is to prevent consumers from thinking that real dairy products are involved. Most nondairy coffee creamers and nondairy whipped toppings contain sodium caseinate.

Some manufacturers go even further, however, and use the label *nondairy* whenever all they have done is to leave out the milk fat. Reduced minerals whey, which, as we'll see later in this chapter, can be very high in lactose, is found in many store-brand nondairy coffee creamers. I've heard of, though not seen, lactose itself included in nondairy products. *Nondairy* can be taken even further, beyond the point of no return. A condensed milk substitute called evaporated mellorine says on its label, "Not a dairy product but a blend of nonfat dairy solids and vegetable oil." The first ingredient on its ingredients list is skimmed milk.

Put bluntly, while the nondairy labeling laws work well to protect the interests of the dairy industry, they are a menace to all of us who cannot have milk. Nondairy products may contain lactose, a problem for the lactose intolerant. Nondairy products with milk proteins can pose a real danger to those with milk allergy. Those who wish to exclude milk for personal or religious reasons can also easily be fooled by products plainly labeled nondairy, which turn out to be no such thing. Reading the fine print on "nondairy" items is an absolute must. Take a look at Chapter 13 to see how to complain to the FDA when you see manufacturers including lactose-containing ingredients in a supposedly nondairy item.

MILK—MASTER OF DISGUISE

Even after you understand how an ingredients list works, you need two more pieces of information before you can intelligently choose whether or not to eat any given product. First, you need to know all the names under which lactose might be hiding in such a listing. Second, you have to know whether each name means an ingredient high or low in lactose.

For example, butter is quite low in lactose. If it's fairly low on the list and no other milk products are listed, it's almost certain that the product as a whole is also low in lactose. Certain dry whey products, on the other hand, can be more than 50 percent lactose. Even very small amounts can contain as much lactose as an eight-ounce glass of milk. Of course, whenever there is more than one source of lactose on a list, you have to worry about their cumulative effect. As a rule of thumb, avoid all products in which you have to add up the lactose content.

In the following pages, I've listed every form, variation, and by-product of milk I've ever come across, along with a description and, where available, an estimated percentage of lactose. These percentages were obtained from a number of sources, resulting in the most comprehensive and complete list I know of. Please read it and refer to it often when you go shopping.

FLUID MILKS

Whole Milk

When the electric guitar came along, the ordinary guitar known for centuries magically acquired the modifier *acoustic* to distinguish it from its amplified descendant. In the same way, plain old everyday milk is called *whole* milk by the dairy people, to separate it from the dozens of variations they have rung on the theme. Whole milk is produced to meet certain minimum legal standards. Once this is done, the final product always contains 4.4 to 4.8 percent lactose.

In ingredients lists, however, the FDA allows concentrated milk, reconstituted milk, and dry whole milk to be listed as *milk*. (To reconstitute a product, you add water to its dry form. Water plus dry whole milk equals reconstituted milk. Reconstituted products will contain about the same amount of lactose as their originals, so reconstituted milk is equal in lactose to whole milk.)

Low-fat Milk

Whole milk must contain, under federal law, not less than 3.25 percent milk fat. If the percentage of milk fat is reduced to 2.0, 1.5, 1.0, or 0.5 percent, the resulting product is low-fat milk. Some low-fat milks have nonfat milk solids added to give them a 10 percent MSNF level, called *protein fortified*. Low-fat milk ranges from 4.8 to 5.5 percent lactose, depending upon the fat content and whether it has been protein fortified.

Skim or Nonfat Milk

When you take as much milk fat away from milk as is technologically possible, the result is skim or nonfat milk (the terms are interchangeable). Skim milk contains 5.1 percent lactose. On an ingredients list, concentrated skim milk, reconstituted skim milk, and nonfat dry milk may be declared skim milk or nonfat milk.

Cream or Light Cream

Technically there is no longer any one product known as cream. *Cream* represents a whole spectrum of high-fat milk products. In everyday usage, however, cream is the same thing as what is formally known as light, coffee, or table cream, any of which must contain between 18 and 30 percent milk fat. Light cream contains 4.2 percent lactose. The FDA says that reconstituted cream, dried cream, and plastic cream (sometimes known as concentrated milk fat) may be called cream on an ingredients listing.

Light Whipping Cream

Whipping cream is heavier than plain light cream, containing between 30 and 36 percent milk fat. Light whipping cream contains 3.6 percent lactose. Whipped cream topping, ready-to-use whipped cream sold in aerosol cans or tubs in stores, is a blend of various milk products. The lactose percentage will vary according to the product, but one figure I've seen is 13.3 percent.

Heavy Cream

Heavy cream is the same as heavy whipping cream. Heavy indeed, it must contain at least 36 percent milk fat. The heavy fat content reduces the lactose content, however, to 3.2 percent.

Half-and-Half

At the other end of the cream spectrum lies half-and-half, a mixture of milk and cream containing between 10.5 and 18 percent milk fat. Half-and-half is the preferred (in taste tests) whitener for coffee. Most restaurants today have moved away from using tiny containers of nondairy creamer and are substituting half-and-half instead. Unfortunately, half-and-half contains 4.5 percent lactose.

Chocolate Milk

Chocolate milk comes in whole, low-fat, and skim varieties. Its lactose content is similar to that of the unflavored milks—about 4.1 to 4.9 percent.

Eggnog

Eggnog is officially a mixture of milk, cream, sugar, milk solids, eggs, stabilizers, and spices, no matter what your Christmas recipe might say. Eggnog-flavored milk, with less milk fat and less egg yolk, is also commercially available. The lactose content of eggnog will vary considerably by recipe but is likely to be in the same range as other fluid milk products.

Low-sodium Milk

Ninety-five percent or more of the sodium in milk can be removed for those people on low-sodium diets. Whole milk is normally used as the starting point. The lactose content is not affected.

CULTURED MILK PRODUCTS

Cultured Buttermilk

Buttermilk is about 4.3 percent lactose. Concentrated sweet cream buttermilk, reconstituted sweet-cream buttermilk, and dried sweet-cream buttermilk may all be described as buttermilk, in those cases when bacterial cultures are not used.

Acidophilus Milk

Acidophilus milk used to be a sour, acid-tasting health food, made by a bacterial culture like those in buttermilk or yogurt.

In recent years, a way of making acidophilus milk without fermentation was devised, resulting in a product with the flavor and consistency of natural milk, but supposedly easier to digest, among other helpful properties. It was even touted as an alternative milk product for those with lactose intolerance, probably because other cultured products, like yogurt, are well tolerated by those with lactose intolerance.

Tests don't provide good evidence of toleration of acidophilus milk. Acidophilus milk seems to have as bad an effect as low-fat milk, probably because the lactose percentage is the same— about 4.9 percent. If you need to have milk, try a lactose-reduced milk instead (discussed in Chapter 7).

Sour Cream

If cream is cultured with bacteria and fermented until the acidity is at least 0.5 percent, the result is sour cream, also called cultured sour cream, containing 3.4 percent lactose. Variations include acidified sour cream, sour half-and-half, and acidified sour half-and-half. If butter is substituted for the cream, sour cream dressing or sour half-and-half dressing appears.

Yogurt

Yogurt is made all over the world, in thousands of individual recipes. In the United States, it is usually commercially made by starting with skim milk and adding about 30 percent milk solids, in the form of nonfat dry milk. This means that the starting material contains 30 percent more protein and calcium—and lactose—than does skim milk. Two types of bacteria are added to ferment the milk mixture. The final product is plain yogurt, which, before it is sweetened or mixed with fruit, is 4.1 percent lactose.

Even many severely intolerant people can eat yogurt with no ill effects, despite its lactose content. For the latest scientific thought on the reasons, see Chapter 7.

CONCENTRATED MILKS

Evaporated Milk

Evaporated milk is a misnomer. In it, milk isn't evaporated but water is—about 60 percent of the milk's water content. What's left is subjected to a complex scheme of homogenizing, standardizing, vitaminizing, stabilizing, and canning. The sealed can is heat treated to sterilize it completely, so that it can sit unopened on a shelf almost indefinitely. Evaporated whole milk contains 9.7 percent lactose. Evaporated skim milk is also available, differing only in that the percentage of milk fat solids is lower.

Concentrated Milk

Concentrated milk is a kind of evaporated milk in which the process has been stopped before the sterilizing stage. This means that concentrated milk will spoil if it is not refrigerated. Very little of it is sold retail. It does, however, contain more lactose than any other variety of fluid milk: 14.7 percent.

Sweetened Condensed Milk

Cans of sweetened condensed milk are not sterilized and yet they can sit on grocery shelves as long as evaporated milk can. How do they do it? With sugar. Lots of sugar; about 40 to 45 percent of the condensed milk; so much that no bacteria can grow in it. Be careful not to confuse evaporated with condensed milk in cooking, as the sugar content in the condensed milk will muck up your recipe unless it is called for specifically. The lactose concentration is high, too—about 11.4 percent.

Dry Milks

Nonfat Dry Milk

If at least 95 percent of the water in skim milk is removed, a powder is formed that is far less bulky, almost as nutritious, and less expensive than fluid milk. Both the standard powdered milks on supermarket shelves and thousands of commercial food products contain nonfat dry milk.

Because so much water is removed, the solids that remain in the dry product are extremely high in lactose—as much as 52.3 percent. The final concentration of lactose depends on the amount of water or other filler added, but it is safe to say that nonfat dry milk appearing high on an ingredients list is a warning sign for anyone with severe lactose intolerance.

Dry Whole Milk

The same process that makes nonfat milk dry can also make powdered whole milk. The lactose content is appreciably lower—about 38.2 percent—although that is still high by ordinary standards.

Butter

Butter

Butter is a combination of milk fat, buttermilk, and water, but mostly fat. Most butter is made from cream, since cream has ten times the butterfat content of milk. Grade AA butter, the best, is made from high-quality fresh sweet cream. This is the grade usually found in supermarkets. Grade A butter is made from fresh cream and Grade B butter from sour cream. In any case, butter has a fat content of over 80 percent.

Since butter is so high in fat, it should be no surprise that it is low in lactose. Estimates vary, but none places the percentage of lactose over 1 percent.

Margarine

All margarines are made of oil and fat, a liquid, emulsifiers, preservatives, artificial butter flavoring, coloring, and added vitamins. If the liquid is plain water, then the margarine probably contains no lactose. Most margarines use a milk product as the liquid. Even so, since margarines, like butter, are 85 percent fat, their lactose percentage is not likely to be very high—almost certainly under 1 percent.

FROZEN MILKS

Ice Cream

Sure, ice cream was once actually made from fresh sweet cream, but today's run-of-the-mill supermarket product may very well use evaporated or powdered milk or even skim milk, and air in amounts varying from near zero to over 50 percent.

As with so many other milk products, all these variations make it difficult to put a firm figure on lactose content. One number I've seen quoted is 6 to 7 percent lactose for plain vanilla ice cream. I'd guess most ordinary flavors run about the same.

Soft Ice Cream, Frozen Custard, and Ice Milk

Nutritionally, soft ice creams aren't much different from their harder counterparts, although they do contain less air and slightly less sugar. Frozen custards, where federal regulations apply, must contain at least 1 percent egg yolks. Even ice cream may be made from milk, so the only real difference between it and ice milk is that the latter is lower in fat than regular ice cream, having a maximum fat content of 7 percent, compared to ice cream's 10 percent. Lactose percentages in these three ice cream variations probably are close to ice cream's estimated 6 to 7 percent, although individual brands may be much higher or lower.

Sherbet

In America, as I explain in Chapter 6, sherbets almost always contain some milk solids along with their fruit flavoring. Low in protein and calcium, sherbet is high only in calories, from the huge amount of sugar (over 1 pound per gallon) added to give it sweetness. United States sherbets run to approximately 2 percent lactose.

Cheeses

Hundreds if not thousands of different cheeses are produced around the world, with most of them available in America's specialty cheese shops. For our purposes, however, we need only set cheese into one of two categories: unripened or ripened.

Unripened Cheeses

All cheeses start with milk. Bacteria and rennin are added next, to sour and thicken the milk. The resulting mixture is warmed until the soft-solid curds separate from the liquid whey. Almost all cheese is made from curds.

Stopping at this point produces most of the familiar soft cheeses. All are fairly high in lactose, because further processing is needed to remove the remaining high-lactose whey. Cream cheese is just under 3 percent lactose, nearly as high as whipping cream. Cottage cheese runs from 2.5 to 3.0 percent lactose, with the 2 percent low-fat variety even higher, at 3.1 to 3.5 percent. Pot cheese and farmer cheese are similar.

Ricotta cheese is a soft, creamy cheese much used in Italian cooking. Unlike most other cheeses, it is made from the whey. I don't have a lactose percentage for it, but its whey content makes ricotta a poor bet for anyone with lactose intolerance, although, again, it may be more suitable for someone allergic to the milk protein, casein.

Ripened Cheeses

The more whey removed from the curds, the firmer the cheese. Once most of the whey is gone, and the lactose with it, cheeses are pressed into molds and aged, or ripened. For example, by law, Cheddar cheese must be aged at least sixty days (unless made from pasteurized milk). Even after two months of aging, a Cheddar is still considered mild. Four to six months of aging produces a medium cheddar, while sharp or extrasharp Cheddars may be aged six to twelve months or even longer.

For all cheeses, the longer the aging, the lower the lactose content. Many eminent authorities say flatly that aging removes all the lactose from cheese, even from cheeses that have only been ripened for a few days. At the same time, I have seen figures for the lactose content of aged Cheddar cheese, as well as Emmentaler and other Swiss cheeses such as Gruyère, that vary from 1.4 to 2.1 percent. Try cheeses cautiously and find your tolerance levels for yourself.

Other cheeses for which I have lactose percentages are American blue, a sharp and usually crumbly cheese, 2.5 percent; Camembert, a semisoft cheese with a crust formed by the mold used to ripen it, 0.4 percent; Gouda, semisoft when young, firmer when aged, 2.1 percent; Edam, something like a skim milk version of Gouda, 1.8 percent; Colby, a variation on Cheddar, 2.5 percent; Parmesan, a good grating cheese, often aged for years in Italy but usually sold when younger in America, 2.9 percent; Stilton, an English cheese, blue-veined from mold, 0.8 percent; and Romadur, a German cheese similar to Limburger, usually served very young, 2.5 percent. To estimate the percentage of lactose in an unfamiliar aged cheese, see if there is any information about its carbohydrate content on the package label. Virtually all the carbohydrate will be lactose. For example, one brand of Swiss cheese claims 0.5 gram of carbohydrate per ounce, or about 1.8 percent lactose.

Most of these cheeses, and most of the others, for that matter, are sold in a number of varieties that have been aged for differing amounts of time. If you're brave enough to try them, always go for the cheeses that have been aged the longest.

Processed Cheese

Several types of processed cheese can be found on the market, each further away from natural cheese than the last. Manufacturers of the first three types that follow must conform to federal standards.

Pasteurized process American cheese is the closest to real cheese, made by grinding Cheddars and adding emulsifiers. The fat and moisture contents must be about the same as the natural cheese from which it is made.

Pasteurized process cheese food can be made with part skim or hard grating cheeses but has less cheese than American cheese does. To make up the difference, other liquid dairy products can be added. But so can water.

Pasteurized process cheese spread must be spreadable at 70 degrees Fahrenheit but can also be made into slices. It has less milk fat and more moisture than a cheese food.

Pasteurized process cheese products have no standard of identity. Although they must be based on dairy products, almost anything else goes, and any additive allowed in foods can be used. Cheese products usually are low fat and low calorie and are aimed at the diet market.

If vegetable oil is substituted for the milk fat, the word *imitation* must be on the label if the product is called cheese. To avoid using the dreaded word *imitation*, some manufacturers simply don't bother to call what they make cheese. Artificially flavored pasteurized process slices are available under a variety of brand names. They contain some cheese but are mostly whey, vegetable oil, and casein.

It's next to impossible to give any meaningful lactose contents for this bizarre array of cheese near-foods. The estimates I've seen range from a minuscule 0.8 percent to a high 7.5 percent. American cheese is likely to be on the low side of this range, however, with the varieties containing whey toward the high end.

WHEY PRODUCTS

Whey

Whey is the liquid left over when the solid curds form in cheese making. Two forms of whey exist: Acid whey has most of its lactose converted into lactic acid. Sweet whey has an insignificant portion of the lactose converted into lactic acid. Guess which form is the one almost exclusively used in commercial foods? (Acid whey does have an occasional use in foods that are already high in acid, like cultured milks.)

Sweet whey (sometimes just called dairy whey) is used so much precisely because it is sweet (being 61 to 75 percent lactose) as well as high in protein (the whey proteins are the second most important milk protein) and relatively inexpensive (being the leftover from an extremely common dairy process).

Whey appears in a confusing hodgepodge of varieties on package labels. Sorting out the lactose percentage of the whey in any individual food is difficult, because many mixtures are possible. In addition, certain varieties of whey do not need to contain a fixed amount of lactose, as long as they are below the maximum fixed by federal law. For example, reduced-lactose whey may be no more than 60 percent lactose, but might be much lower in a particular product. Please keep that in mind when you see the following astoundingly high percentages. You should also keep in mind that concentrated whey, reconstituted whey, and dried whey may be declared simply as *whey* on ingredient lists.

Concentrated Whey

Removing some of the liquid in whey, without changing the relative proportions of anything else, results in concentrated whey. Concentrated whey, therefore, has the same lactose percentage as regular liquid whey; 61 to 75 percent.

Dry Whey

Dry whey is concentrated whey with all the water removed, but again all the other constituents in the same relative proportions. It, too, has the same lactose percentage: 61 to 75 percent.

Reduced-Lactose Whey

Well, *reduced* is a relative term. The lactose content of reduced-lactose whey cannot exceed 60 percent, if that's any comfort to you. This variation can also come in fluid, concentrated, or dry form.

Reduced-Minerals Whey

Ash is the nonorganic component of foods, which mostly means minerals. Whey normally has 7 to 14 percent ash, but reduced-minerals whey is limited to 7 percent ash. The difference seems to be made up with lactose since, with the exception of pure lactose itself, reduced-minerals whey has the highest lactose content of any milk product—up to a maximum of 85 percent lactose. A variant is partially demineralized whey solids.

Whey Protein Concentrate

From boosting the protein level to a minimum of 25 percent, whey becomes whey protein concentrate. It may come in liquid, concentrated, or dry forms. Whichever way it comes, it can be no more than 60 percent lactose.

Dried Dairy Blend

A combination of whey and the milk protein calcium caseinate, the lactose content of dried dairy blend will vary with the blender but is probably high.

Milk Solids

Milk solids include the protein, carbohydrate (lactose), fat, vitamins, and minerals, in short, everything in milk but the water. Solids of one sort or another are commonly added to food. I've seen milk solids, skim milk solids, buttermilk solids, sour cream solids, butter solids, and whey solids, but other variations undoubtedly exist. All are likely to be similar in lactose content to the dry version of the same form.

Milk Proteins

Milk doesn't contain an enormous amount of protein—only about 3.3 percent on the average—but it is very high quality protein, furnishing all the amino acids essential for nutrition and many others besides.

Most of the milk protein—some 82 percent—comes from casein, a family of related proteins. Casein concentrates in the curds from which cheese is formed, making cheese a higher protein food than milk itself. In fact, many food processors throw a little casein into their products so that the numbers on the nutrition label look higher than they otherwise would. Casein also makes imitation products work more like the real thing and so is often included in so-called nondairy products.

Is it dangerous? For the lactose intolerant, probably not. Casein comes from milk, and so it's possible—even likely—that a few molecules of lactose may have tagged along with it, but the chance of these affecting anyone with lactose intolerance is small. Some of the sodium caseinate–containing nondairy products even say *lactose-free* on their labels. Of course, people with milk protein allergies should stay far away from everything with casein, no matter that it says *nondairy* on the outside.

The remaining 18 percent of the milk protein comes out of the whey portion. Here two families predominate: the lactalbumins and the lactoglobulins. One form of the latter, beta-lactoglobulin, can cause even worse allergic reactions than casein. Oddly enough, while the lactose and casein in goat's milk are similar to that of cow's milk, the whey proteins are not. If you're sure you have only the whey protein allergy, then you might want to take a chance on goat's milk for a change of pace.

For those of us who are lactose intolerant, goat's milk is out, but we're probably safe if the pure proteins lactalbumin or lactoglobulin appear by themselves on a product label. Remember, whey protein concentrate is not a pure protein but merely a high-protein version of whey, and very high in lactose.

Hydrolyzed milk protein is protein that has been treated to make it less allergenic. It is found in many products, including some infant formulas.

MILK FATS

Most milk fat products are low in lactose, if they contain any at all. Butter, which I've already mentioned, is 85 percent milk fat and only a fraction of a percent lactose. Butter is sometimes disguised in foods as butter solids or natural butter flavor, and of course most margarines contain some milk fat.

Pure fats—milk fat, butterfat, and butter oil—are also sometimes added to foods. All are likely to be virtually lactose free. Both butter oil and anhydrous butterfat may be referred to as butterfat on ingredients listings, by the way.

Very occasionally you may see a milk fat identified by one of its chemical names. With over five hundred different fatty acids identified in milk, there is no way to list them all here. Fortunately, they fall into a few large families. Saturated fatty acids include myristic acid, palmitic acid, and stearic acid. Unsaturated fatty acids include oleic acid, linoleic acid, and linolenic acid. Any of these or their variations (sodium stearyl lactylate and glycerol lacto palmitate are two I've actually seen on food labels) probably are safe.

Other

Imitation and Filled Milk

Combining water, vegetable oil, fish protein, corn syrup solids, and some miscellaneous milk products like casein, whey, or lactose can produce a fluid that looks a lot like milk. If it isn't as nutritious as milk itself, however, then it must be called imitation milk.

Removing the milk fat from whole milk, low-fat milk, light cream, or half-and-half and replacing it with a fat or oil from another source gives you filled milk. It is also not as nutritious as the original product.

Both imitation milk and filled milk are quite rare nowadays. I have never seen either included on any ingredients listing. The wide variation in the way they can be made makes it impossible to give a lactose percentage. You should be aware, if you ever stumble across them, that the American Academy of Pediatrics considers imitation and filled milk products inappropriate for feeding infants and young children.

Lactic Acid

Lactic acid is what the bacteria in cultured milk products turn lactose into. For this reason, lactic acid is lactose-free. It appears in ingredients lists every once in a while, causing endless confusion, but by itself, it is perfectly safe.

ESTIMATED PERCENTAGE OF LACTOSE IN MILK PRODUCTS

FLUID MILKS

whole milk	4.4–4.8
low-fat milk	4.8–5.5
skim or nonfat milk	4.9–5.1
light cream	4.0–4.2
light whipping cream	3.6
whipped cream topping	13.3
heavy cream	3.2
half-and-half	4.0–4.2
chocolate milk	4.1–4.9

CULTURED MILK PRODUCTS

buttermilk	3.7–4.7
acidophilus milk	4.9
sour cream	3.4
yogurt (from whole milk)	4.1–4.8
yogurt (milk solids added)	6.6

CONCENTRATED MILKS

evaporated milk	9.7
concentrated milk	14.7
sweetened condensed milk	11.4

DRY MILKS

nonfat dry milk	35.9–52.3
dry whole milk	37.5–38.2

BUTTER

butter	0.3–1.0
margarine	0.0–1.0

FROZEN MILKS

ice cream (vanilla)	6.8
ice milk (vanilla)	7.5
sherbet (orange)	2.1

CHEESES

unripened cheeses

cream cheese	2.9
cottage cheese	2.5–3.0
cottage cheese (2% fat)	3.1–3.5

ripened cheeses

Cheddar	1.4–2.1
American blue	2.5
Camembert	0.4
Gouda	2.1
Edam	1.8
Parmesan	2.9
Stilton	0.8
Romadur	2.5
Colby	2.5

processed cheeses

American	1.8
process cheese food	7.5

WHEY

whey	61–75
concentrated whey	61–75

dry whey   61–75
reduced lactose whey   maximum 60
reduced minerals whey   maximum 85
whey protein concentrate   maximum 60

MILK SOLIDS

PROTEINS

casein, sodium caseinate, calcium caseinate   0.0
lactalbumins, lactoglobulins   0.0

FATS

milk fat, butterfat, butter oil   0.0

OTHER

lactic acid   0.0

CHAPTER SIX

THE LACTOSE-FREE DIET

This chapter is dedicated to the proposition that all milk is created equal—and that it's all bad for you. Every single food containing lactose has the potential for causing unpleasant symptoms, and few people ever eat just one milk product in the course of a day. They're eaten in combination, or in sequence, or in dribs and drabs from morning till night, with lactose piling up in the system each time.

Even people with mild lactose intolerance may find that they have to cut back on their normal consumption of milk products to stay within their tolerance limit. Severely lactose-intolerant individuals have no choice; they need to learn all the substitutes they can. And don't forget, the majority of those diagnosed as lactose intolerant by specialists are placed on lactose-free diets.

So for the rest of this chapter, forget there ever was such a thing as milk. No half measures. Manufacturers make substitutes for milk, cream, butter, ice cream, whipped cream, cream cheese, and sour cream, every one of them completely lactose free. Some are closer to the original than others (and not everyone agrees which these are: personal tastes play a great role in deciding the acceptability of these substitutes). Not all of them are available everywhere in the country, either. The East Coast has far greater variety in its milk substitutes than do the Midwest or West Coast.

Every day more and more people are demanding lactose-free products, and manufacturers are listening. Even the ones who put out milk-free products not specifically for the lactose-intolerant market find that putting the words *lactose free* on their packages increases their sales. Support these milk substitutes. Let your local stores know that you want them, and write and tell the manufacturers why you're buying their products. If we convince them that a truly sizable market exists, we'll continue to see our choices expand year after year.

The rest of this chapter describes in detail the substitutes I'm aware of. Once you know about these, you may be able to find even more in your local stores. A few words of caution for when you go out on your own:

- "Imitation" products are not always the same as milk substitutes. Imitation sour cream, for example, has milk products in it. The FDA requires manufacturers to label a product *imitation* if it is similar to but not as nutritious as the original.
- "Nondairy" products can contain milk-derived ingredients, including some that contain lactose.
- Casein, calcium caseinate, and sodium caseinate are milk proteins that are often added to foods (including many "nondairy" foods). It's highly unlikely that any of these proteins will contain lactose. In fact, some of the substitutes I'll mention that label themselves lactose free include sodium caseinate. However, people with milk protein allergy should definitely stay away from casein or any of its derivatives. For those people with lactose intolerance who want to be especially cautious, and for those who have other reasons for avoiding milk, I will point out the presence of sodium caseinate in any of the milk substitutes, and I will favor substitutes that are completely free of any milk-derived ingredients.

Milk and Cream Substitutes

Need a milk substitute? Try water. Cheap, easily available, and basically healthy, water can be substituted directly for milk in a host of recipes. Tastes great on a hot summer day, too.

In fact, for a lot of recipes, almost anything liquid will do— orange juice, the syrup from a can of fruit, even beer. Sure, the final taste will vary some, but isn't that half the goal in experimenting in the kitchen?

Milk, admittedly, is more than just a liquid. Its fat content is a necessity in many recipes and is just as necessary for helping the body use the fat-soluble vitamins A, D, E, and K. Milk (or cream) whips, sets in puddings and custards, and gives body to foods. And yes, it tastes great on a hot summer day. Any other time, too.

No milk substitute will give you all that. Two are very close, however, and have a few other advantages as well. Both are easily found in supermarkets, mix well in coffee, and are even colored white. In other ways, they couldn't be less alike, one being a mass of "chemicals" and the other a "natural" product, though these distinctions may be more apparent than real. I'm referring to the nondairy creamers and the soy milks.

NONDAIRY CREAMERS

Powdered nondairy creamers won their way into the coffee cups of America by way of the office coffee machine. With no handy refrigerator to pull a bottle of milk or cream from, the millions of caffeine addicts who demanded their coffee light were in a bind. They needed a product that would perform cream's most important function—cutting the bitterness of coffee—while being able to last indefinitely sitting on a shelf. Most people will accept the taste of a powdered creamer, but to get the powder to work the same way as cream, the manufacturers had to cheat. Virtually all the powdered "nondairy" creamers on the market contain sodium caseinate.

As general, all-purpose milk substitutes, the powdered nondairy creamers don't work as well as the liquid nondairy creamers. With one major exception—Mocha Mix, found only on the West Coast—the liquid creamers are all to be found in the frozen food section of the supermarket. (Mocha Mix comes refrigerated.) The dominant national brand is Coffee Rich, with so much of the market that it doesn't even have any regional competition. Most supermarkets have their own private label or house brand frozen creamer, manufactured by a variety of companies.

The following information refers and applies specifically to Coffee Rich, since it is the one product you're all likely to run into. Feel free to experiment with the house brand at your favorite store.

When thawed for a day or so in the refrigerator, Coffee Rich turns into a thick white liquid. It will last a year frozen, two to three weeks thawed in the refrigerator. Once out of the refrigerator, Coffee Rich doesn't last very long at all—no more than four hours at room temperature—so be careful. If you forget and leave it out overnight, toss it.

Poured straight out of the container, Coffee Rich will substitute for cream or half-and-half in coffee or in baking. The high fat content (about 10½ to 11 percent) makes it unsuitable for a straight milk substitute. When the recipe calls for a milk substitute, use the following guidelines:

FOR	USE
1 cup milk	½ cup Coffee Rich and ½ cup water
1 cup skim milk	2 ounces Coffee Rich and 6 ounces water
1 cup half-and-half	1 cup Coffee Rich
1 cup cream	1 cup Coffee Rich
1 cup sweetened condensed milk	1 cup Coffee Rich
1 cup buttermilk	1 tablespoon vinegar and enough Coffee Rich to make 1 cup

Because Coffee Rich lacks milk protein, it won't "set" in custards and puddings. Adding cornstarch as a thickener will help, but the end result is still not the same. With these exceptions, go back to your favorite cookbook and start experimenting with all the recipes you thought you would never use again. Coffee Rich will even heat and reheat three times with acceptable results, although it should not be boiled for long periods.

One of the admitted problems of Coffee Rich and most other

liquid nondairy creamers is that coconut oil is used to supply the necessary fat content (though see the section on Mocha Mix, p. 100). Coconut oil is one of the most highly saturated fats available, even more so than milk fat. Ever since saturated fats were identified as possible contributors to heart disease, many people have been placed on a low-saturated-fat diet. On such a diet, you're supposed to avoid whole milk, butter, fatty meats, egg yolks, and potato chips, among other foods, and stick to foods containing polyunsaturated fats.

Where there's a market, there's a product; most liquid nondairy creamer manufacturers also make a milk substitute that uses polyunsaturated fats in place of the coconut oil. The polyunsaturated equivalent to Coffee Rich is called, unsurprisingly, Poly Rich. It tests out to about the same level of saturation as sunflower-seed oil, low on the saturation scale. Poly Rich has a considerably different taste than Coffee Rich, something like skim milk to Coffee Rich's whole milk. The fat content is from 100 percent soybean oil, which imparts a bean-y taste that is not to many people's liking. In baking, however, it works exactly as Coffee Rich does; just substitute one for the other whenever you want to drop the saturated-fat content of your food. Poly Rich is available nationally, but not all food wholesalers handle it. If you can't find it, try asking your local supermarket to obtain it. Many supermarkets are willing to help with special orders, especially if you can convince them that you're not the only one interested in the product.

In my local supermarket, early in 1986, Coffee Rich sold for about forty-five cents for the 16 ounce (1 pound) size. One quart of whole milk runs about eighty-nine cents. Since one pound of Coffee Rich diluted with an equal amount of water is the equivalent in cooking of about a quart of whole milk, Coffee Rich is considerably cheaper. It is *not* nutritionally equal, lacking the calcium and many of the vitamins of milk. Calcium supplements are a necessity on a milk-free diet (more on this in Chapter 10).

When traveling, it's nice to know that Coffee Rich is distributed internationally. Canada has it, England distributes it to continental Europe, and it can also be found in Hong Kong, Japan, and Australia.

Closer to home, if you're ever traveling to Buffalo, be sure to stop at Rich's Outlet Store, at 1150 Niagara Street, Buffalo NY 14270 (which is also the Rich Products Corporation mailing address). Here you can buy all sorts of their institutional products that are not available retail, including bags of the restaurant-size Coffee Rich individual serving containers (plus the sodium caseinate–containing powdered Coffee Rich) and Rich's Bettercreme nondairy icing and filling, along with other Rich products and a store full of definitely unsafe bakery items. Many of the items in the Outlet Store are normally aimed at institutions and so come in packages far too huge to be useful to an individual. You could share with your lactose-intolerant friends, though, and the frozen products have extremely long lives if kept frozen.

Mocha Mix

Mocha Mix doesn't have the national distribution that Coffee Rich does—it's only available in California, Washington, Oregon, and Arizona—but westerners are sure to be familiar with it.

Unlike all the other liquid nondairy creamers I've seen, Mocha Mix comes "fresh"—that is, refrigerated—rather than frozen. It also comes completely free of cholesterol and is low in calories and in saturated fats. Using partially hydrogenated soybean oil in place of coconut or palm kernel oils is the secret of this healthiness.

Mocha Mix is made by Presto Food Products, Inc., 929 East 14th Street, Los Angeles, CA 90021.

SOY MILKS

Soy is fashionable. In America, that is. In the Far East, soy has been a staple in the diet for thousands of years, and for very good reason. Soybeans are 35 percent protein, more than other unprocessed food. Soy protein even contains all eight essential amino acids needed by the body, very unusual for plant protein. Soy contains no cholesterol, is low in saturated fats, is extremely inexpensive, and can be transformed into foods that themselves are the basis for hundreds of recipes. Tofu, miso (fermented soybean paste), shoyu (soy sauce), and tempeh (fermented soybean cakes) are all beginning to move out of the import stores and gourmet sections onto regular supermarket shelves and restaurant menus. And the push is on to add tonyu—soy milk—to the list.

Soybeans would have long since conquered the world if it weren't for the inarguable fact that soybeans tend to taste like soybeans, and most Westerners don't like the taste at all. Modern food technology has sprung to the rescue, much to the dismay of the soy purists, and has succeeded in producing soy-based foods that are salable in the United States.

At present, then, there are two types of soy milk. One is homemade or sold in small quantities at natural foods stores, extremely inexpensive, healthy, "natural," and for a distinctly minority audience. The other is a commercial product, sweetened, flavored, milder, and enjoying booming sales.

I emphasize the word *commercial*. *Natural* simply doesn't apply to a product that has been vacuum de-aerated, vacuum deodorized, homogenized, centrifuged, dehulled, superheated, and has had its enzymes deactivated, all in an airtight container that can last for a month on a shelf with no refrigeration. Commercial soy milk is definitely a processed food.

Although the United States grows its own soybeans, very few of them are processed in this country. Instead, most are exported to Japan for conversion into soy milk, which happens to involve adding large quantities of water. You pay five times as much for commercial soy milk as you do for cow's milk because you're paying to have Japanese water shipped across the Pacific Ocean.

No one company dominates the commercial soy milk market the way Coffee Rich dominates the liquid nondairy creamer market. Hundreds of small and medium-size companies, some local, some in China, Hong Kong, and Japan, distribute some variety of soy milk. A few products have led the way in opening the soy milk market to a national audience. These include Eden's Edensoy, Great Eastern Sun's Ah Soy, Westbrae's Westsoy and Malteds (all made in Japan); Health Valley Natural Food's Soy Moo (made in the United States and in Belgium); and Hong Kong Soya Bean Products' Vitasoy. All come in plain and flavored forms. Some come both frozen and in what the food industry calls brik-paks, those nonrefrigerated serving-size boxes used for a number of juices and other beverages.

The major commercial soy milks use a process developed by researchers at Cornell University (and refined by Japanese scientists) that lessens the bean-y taste of the drink. Although the processing, along with the added sugar, reduces the nutritiousness of the product, soy milk still contains more protein, less fat, and more iron and niacin than does cow's milk, all without cholesterol.

For all this, soy milk is still something of an acquired taste. Not that the commercial varieties taste bad. Plain soy milk, in fact, doesn't have much of a taste at all, although for some people, its aftertaste can be lingering and unpleasant. As a bland, white liquid, soy milk is useful as a milk substitute in baking without adding extra flavor to the finished product.

Homemade soy milk is a very different product, although it is at least as versatile. It can be served hot or cold, plain, sweetened, or with added fruit. The cost is far, far less than that of the commercial varieties, and less than a quarter of the cost of cow's milk.

Both varieties of soy milk will make yogurt, milkshakes, or whipped "cream." Unlike Coffee Rich, soy milk can be used in making custards and puddings. I've seen recipes for pancakes, waffles, and mousse, and if you checked through enough soy cookbooks, you'd probably find recipes for cakes and cookies.

Making soy milk looks complicated at first, involving soaking the beans, grinding them, making a puree, and then boiling the liquid you press from the puree until it is the desired thickness, equivalent to milk or cream. Once the liquid is drawn off, you can make tofu with the remaining paste. Numerous recipes exist for making soy milk; too many to get into here. Probably the best book on the subject is William Shurtleff and Akiko Aoyagi's *The Book of Tofu*, which is knowledgeable, exhaustive, and enthusiastic. If you want to make soy milk using the Cornell process to change the taste, I recommend instead *The Tofu Cookbook*, by Cathy Bauer and Juel Anderson, which is far more oriented toward American eating habits. Dozens of other books on tofu, tempeh, and the whole gamut of soy-based products are now available at mainstream bookstores, allowing you your choice of a level of purism.

Soy Milk Formulas

Canned commercial soy milks abound in the baby food section of the supermarket, in formulas designed to substitute for human or cow's milk for those babies who cannot tolerate them. They can also be used to make foods for adults, just as the other milk substitutes can, and the formula companies produce cookbooks to prove it. Addresses for these cookbooks are in Chapter 12, and more details on the formulas themselves are in Chapter 9.

BUTTER SUBSTITUTES

The magnificently named Hippolyte Mege-Mouries, a French chemist, produced his first batch of oleomargarine in the 1860s. Emperor Napoleon III had offered a prize for the best substitute for butter, which had become extremely expensive, was sometimes adulterated with lard, and turned rancid easily. Mege-Mouries extracted oleo oil from beef fat, blended it with chopped cow's bladder, added a blend of fats called margarin, and churned the mixture with milk and water.

Today the oleo is gone from margarine and so is the chopped cow's bladder. Unfortunately, most margarines have kept the milk in some form, and those margarines are as much a problem as is butter for the lactose intolerant.

Margarines come hard, as sticks; soft, in tubs; and liquid, in squeezable bottles, with further distinctions in each category, the most important of which are the salted and unsalted varieties. Regular margarines are, like butter, at least 80 percent fat, with most of the rest being water. More water can easily be blended to produce a product with less fat and fewer calories: light margarine spreads have 50 to 60 percent fat, while diet margarines have only 40 percent fat, with that much more water. The fat content can come from corn, cottonseed, peanut, sunflower, safflower, or soybean oil. (One margarine, which calls itself safflower oil margarine on the front of the box, also includes soybean oil and partially hydrogenated soybean and cottonseed oils in its list of ingredients.) The one great blessing of all this confusing variation is that, almost certainly, you can find a milk-free margarine that is right for you.

One of the odd facts about milk-free margarines is that so many of them—like Fleischmann's and Mazola—only come in an unsalted form (sometimes called sweet unsalted, to imitate the sweet unsalted butters). Others, however, including kosher margarines like Mother's and Manischewitz, and specialty products like Hain Safflower Oil Margarine, come both salted and unsalted. Don't assume that every unsalted margarine will also be milk free, though; read the label carefully.

All the margarines I just listed, along with their salted cousins like Nucoa and Shedd's Willow Run Soy Bean Margarine, are regular stick margarines, which are the best for baking and frying. (Leaving out the milk actually improves margarine for frying, since unsalted milk-free margarine won't turn brown or burn in the pan as fast as margarines with milk.) Milk-free soft varieties, such as Nucoa Soft, are the best for actually spreading onto breads, rolls, and muffins. Stick margarines need two to four hours out of the refrigerator for equal spreadability.

Some of the kosher margarines come every which way. Mother's, for example, has salted and unsalted stick versions as well as salted and unsalted soft margarines. Though these kosher specialty brands may be harder to find in your area, their versatility makes them worth the search.

Light spreads create a nice middle ground between the full-calorie and diet margarines. Lower in fat and calories and, as their name implies, easier to spread than the sticks, they are still usable in cooking. A glob of a light spread, though tough to measure, melts more rapidly than a block of a stick margarine, a plus for doing some quick cooking. The better spreads also compare very favorably to the regular margarines in taste, with some people actually preferring them. Well-known milk-free spreads include Parkay Light Spread, Mrs. Filbert's Family Spread, and Shedd's Spread Country Crock (although Shedd's sticks are *not* milk free).

A number of margarines leave out the high-calorie milk products in their quest for diet status, including Imperial Diet and Diet Imperial Imitation, Weight Watchers Reduced Calorie (which comes in sticks, and salted and unsalted soft varieties), Blue Bonnet Diet, and Mazola Diet Reduced Calorie. Diet margarines shouldn't be used at all for baking or frying. Their reduced fat content makes it impossible to substitute them one-for-one with butter. Using them may make baked foods tough or cause fried foods to stick to the pan or cook unevenly. Diet margarines also tend to taste no better than they bake, while the full-calorie stick margarines have fooled more than half the people in blind taste tests against butter. Unless you have a desperately urgent need to cut down on calories or are on a totally fat-controlled diet, I'd recommend against any of the diet margarines.

Margarines, like other dairy products, are often sold only regionally. As always, my advice is to read all the labels of all the margarines your supermarket sells. Other good places to find milk-free margarines are in health food stores and in kosher delicatessens.

ICE CREAM SUBSTITUTES

Writing about frozen nondairy desserts is a little like writing about computers back in the early 1980s. So much is happening, with old companies constantly expanding and new companies coming onto the market seemingly every day, that almost anything I say will be obsolete by the time you read this. So take the following old news about specific brand names with a grain of salt—or a dollop of hot fudge—in the hope that none of the basics will change, and then go out and enjoy all the new products that debuted on the market after I wrote this.

Imitation ice creams have been around for years, especially for the kosher market, those who can't or won't mix meat and milk at the same meal (see the section on pareve foods in Chapter 8). For the same number of years, imitation ice creams were terrible. And then came tofu: high in protein, low in saturated-fat, low in calories, milk-free tofu, the far eastern food that inventive Westerners can make imitate anything. David Mintz, owner of a kosher restaurant and catering service, decided that tofu was perfect for the frozen dessert his customers wanted. The customers waited almost ten years while Mintz threw away thousands of failed experimental batches, but in the end, he brought forth Tofutti, and a fad was born.

Tofutti wasn't the first—Ice Bean has been around since 1976—but its great taste and Mintz's promotional savvy made it a must in trendy New York, which caused the fad to spread to the rest of the country. Tofutti comes in two versions—a soft serve whipped out of a machine, and a hard pack for supermarkets. Häagen-Dazs, the big name in high-end ice cream, is distributing Tofutti through its nationwide chain of stores. Flavors include wildberry, vanilla-almond bark, and peanut butter.

Not to be outdone, Frusen Gladje, Häagen-Dazs's rival, is bankrolling Gloria Vanderbilt's (I told you, trendy) Glacé Tofu Frozen Dessert. It was such a hit upon its introduction in 1985 that the company immediately added a whole line of products, including a Fruit 'N Creme Bar, a Cookie 'N Creme Sandwich, and an Orange Creme Treat, all similarly lactose free.

Shopping around always produces a few names not backed by huge national corporations and their advertising budgets. Some of the ones I've seen or read about are the previously mentioned Ice Bean, Parvelle, Tofait, Penguino's (which claims to use 20 percent tofu in its recipe, as opposed to as little as 3 percent in some of its rivals), and Gourmet Tofu by Riviera. Mocha Mix also makes a line of seven flavors of Non-Dairy Frozen Dessert. Phoenix Foods' Ta-Tou Lite, introduced in Philadelphia, claims to be the first "light" tofu product. On the West Coast, McQueen's Natural Dairy-Free Frozen Dessert, distributed in California and Hawaii, includes calcium in the form of oyster shells, just like a mineral supplement. Even before Gloria, Tuscan Dairy Farms, in New Jersey, introduced Tofu Bars, supposedly the first tofu product on a stick. Not all these actually list tofu as an ingredient, although they all use soybeans. Some of the largest national food corporations, having noted the success of Tofutti, are now making plans for frozen desserts of their own. Perhaps in a few years, a tofu-based product will be a must at every ice cream stand in the country.

Trendy or not, the burning question is, how do they taste? Well, of all the milk substitutes I've tried, none come closer to the real thing than the frozen tofu desserts. Slightly lighter than ice cream, they nonetheless have a full rich taste in a variety of delicious flavors. The soft serve works well in a cone, and the hard pack makes a superb sundae. Try some with loganberry syrup for a treat you won't find in an ice cream parlor.

Many of the products are being marketed specifically as lactose-free desserts, though they're obviously being bought by nearly everyone. A superior and milk-free product, they're helping set the course for other substitute products aimed at the lactose in-tolerant, a market big enough to cater to. It's hard not to cheer for their success.

RICE DREAM

Tofu isn't the only traditional Japanese product to invade the ice cream market. Beyond tofu lies amasake, a nondairy milk made in a culturing process from brown rice. Imagine Foods, out of Fayetteville, Arkansas, turns amasake into Rice Dream. Rice Dream comes in the usual variety of flavors, always substituting carob for chocolate in the best health-food tradition, and in both pints and soft serve.

There's no getting around the fact that Rice Dream is simply different from the tofu-based desserts, with a taste all its own. I can't resist quoting the list of ingredients from the carob chip flavor:

> Well water, chico-san brown rice, koji (cultured) rice, chico-san rice syrup, sesami tahini, Vermont grade A maple syrup, unsweetened milk-free carob chips, vanilla, extracts from Irish moss and guar beans, sea salt.

SORBETS, ICES, AND SORBUTTI

Most places that carry ice cream also carry sherbet, but in America, milk is almost invariably an ingredient in sherbet. Only a few kosher specialty lines manufacture nondairy sherbet, although if you're ever in my home town of Rochester, New York, stop in at Abbott's Frozen Custard for an unbelievably good sherbet that looks and tastes as if it contains milk but somehow doesn't.

In Europe, the French and Italians take a different tack. They mix uncooked pureed fruit and a cooked sugar-water syrup to make fruit ices bursting with fresh fruit flavor. The French call theirs a sorbet, while the Italians have the very similar *sorbetti* and also *granite*, which is closer in texture to Sno-Kones. Be warned that the Italian ices are sometimes called gelato, a name that in this country usually applies only to a heavy, egg yolk– based variety of ice cream. All the fruit ices, along with a true sugarless frozen ice, can easily be made at home. Most of the so-called women's magazines feature recipes in every year's summer issues.

Part of the American way is to take everything that can be made at home and turn it into a commercial extravaganza. Two sorbets heading for the national market—Le Sorbet, distributed by the ever-busy Häagen-Dazs, and Castle & Cooke's Dole Fruit Sorbet—are receiving heavy advertising in test markets. Sorbets have extremely intense fruit flavors that can be shocking at first bite; they taste nothing like the blander American sherbets. Sorbet flavors are also more exotic. Le Sorbet is packaging seven, including mango, cassis, and passion fruit, and has more than thirty flavors in its stores.

Before we get too exotic, remember that the lowly Popsicle is also a milk-free frozen fruit–flavored dessert. Jell-O has even come out with several flavors of frozen gelatin, also milk free. The Eskimo Pie people now make Welch's Frozen Grape Juice Bars and Minute Maid Frozen Orange Juice Bars. Frozfruit makes delicious frozen fruit bars in a variety of flavors, although some do contain milk, including the banana and coconut. And so on, and so on. Ices don't seem ready to take away the market from ice cream, but they will always be with us.

WHIPPED CREAM SUBSTITUTES

If you've ever whipped cream, you know that it needs to be used immediately; you can't let it sit around overnight. Many restaurants and big institutional cafeterias can't be bothered to whip up expensive cream every time someone wants a topping. They'd much rather make up one big batch early in the day, put it on the puddings and pies, and let the desserts just sit there until somebody buys them. Only nondairy substitutes have this appealing character.

One of these, Richwhip, made by the makers of Coffee Rich, is now available in stores in certain areas. Richwhip comes frozen, in half-pint containers. To use it, thaw, shake well, and then whip at medium speed just like whipping cream. It produces a greater volume of whipped topping than an equivalent amount of the real thing, and it won't break down overnight. Richwhip can sit in the refrigerator for two months, if unopened, and for a year in the freezer; another advantage over cream. If it is not carried in your area, you might try looking in the Yellow Pages for a food wholesaler that carries Rich's products for the institutional market.

Far more common and readily available are the ready-to-use whipped toppings. The big national brand is Cool Whip, the omnipresent whipped topping in a tub, star of countless desserts and gelatin molds. Cool Whip and its competitors come frozen and stay nicely in the freezer for long periods of time. To use, let thaw a good six hours in the refrigerator. These products can be refrozen, which is necessary since they last only about two weeks in the refrigerator once they're opened. Thawed, the whipped toppings are easy to spoon onto anything you care to use them on and have a fine, rich taste. Cool Whip does contain sodium caseinate.

The people who make Mocha Mix also produce a nondairy whipped topping of their own, called dsertwhip, funny spelling and all.

With the new trend toward naturalness in food, most of the manufacturers are putting out varieties of whipped toppings that do contain cream and other milk products. Why aren't they called whipped creams, then? Because the first ingredient is skim milk. Be careful when reading labels so you don't get fooled by them.

A few aerosol cans of whipped topping are still available, including Richwhip Non-Dairy Whipped Topping. As a kid, I thought one of the great treasures in life was getting to squeeze the aerosol nozzle to smother a dessert in mounds of crinkly toppings. A variation, Rich's Whipped Topping, which contains sodium caseinate, comes in an applicator bag, with a fluted tip to make fancy decorations. Again, aerosol cans of real whipped cream are easy to find. What you want to look for is whipped topping.

One further completely milk-free Rich product that is only available institutionally or at the Rich's Outlet Store is Rich's Bettercreme filling and icing. Like Richwhip, Bettercreme whips up to make a filling for donuts and pastries and between layers of cakes or as an icing. It lasts a year in the freezer or six months in the refrigerator, and comes in chocolate and vanilla flavors. Again, try a local food wholesaler to see if this might be available in your area.

Other Substitutes

The only cream cheese substitute I know of is King Smoothie Imitation Cream Cheese, made by American Whipped Products of Newburgh, New York. Smoothie is one of a line of imitation milk products, all with names beginning with King. It is the only one that is lactose free.

Originally introduced merely as a lower-calorie, low-fat imitation cream cheese, Smoothie's sales picked up when people discovered it was also lactose free, which is now proclaimed right on the label (although it does include sodium caseinate). Because of the lower fat content, Smoothie can't be considered a perfect substitute. Baking is especially a problem. You'll have to experiment to discover exactly how to substitute it in any hot dishes. It works fine cold and makes a good interface between bagels and lox.

Smoothie is another product pretty much restricted to the East Coast, although it is sold in a few places in California.

Maybe in the future, every milk product will have a substitute easily available, but if you want to go beyond the ones I've already mentioned, you'll have to go out and really search. Kosher delis are the best place to find individual, odd milk substitutes, since they're the only consistent market the manufacturers know of.

In them, I've found Heller's imitation sour cream, a milk-free product that makes a passable beef stroganoff. I also once found a completely milk-free cheese substitute, which I won't mention by name since I haven't seen it on the market for years. I'll never know how it tasted. It looked and smelled so bad I never got up the courage to take a single bite.

Major centers of the Jewish market, like New York City, probably have a better selection of such items than elsewhere in the country, but kosher delis are spotted everywhere. They have much in them for the lactose intolerant, and I urge you to search them out for yourselves. (More on kosher and pareve foods can be found in Chapter 8.)

HEY, FRED, WHERE'S THE POWDERED SOY MILK?

A problem with all these milk substitutes is that few of them are likely to be carried at your corner convenience store. To find the greatest number of them you need a supermarket, the larger the better.

Because no organized group has been demanding and buying them, none of the milk substitutes I've been talking about falls into the fast-moving, large-selling category. Consequently they get shoved into any old corner of the store that doesn't have better things to push at you. At first, shopping for milk substitutes may be a long and tedious experience as you march up and down the miles of aisles in a superstore searching for products you've never heard of before. Quick, tell me—where would you think to look for frozen, refrigerated, and powdered soy milks? Why aren't the frozen nondairy whipped toppings near the frozen nondairy coffee creamers? Why are there entire aisles full of cat and dog food but three packages of pareve margarine in the kosher section?

Learning to psych out the merchandising strategy of your local supermarket manager is a skill you may never have thought you needed to master, but it's as important for your peace of mind as learning to adapt your recipes. Some consumer pressure for getting a larger number or wider variety of milk-free products in the store also wouldn't hurt. (More discussion of consumer politics for the lactose intolerant is in Chapter 13.)

CHAPTER SEVEN

THE LACTOSE-REDUCED DIET

Nobody knows exactly how many millions of Americans have lactose intolerance: the estimates grow higher each year. But you can be sure that if all of you—all 25 million or 30 million or 50 million—could have no milk, our whole commercial food industry would be different. Supermarkets would be filled with milk substitutes, restaurants would have special menus, pills and nostrums would flood the drugstores.

We may yet see this. There's certainly no shortage of stomach ailments in this country, and as awareness of lactose intolerance grows, more and more people will surely realize that their chronic discomfort is nothing more than an inability to digest lactose. Some will join the ranks of those who should never touch milk or milk products. The rest of you need to be able to answer a crucial question—how much lactose is safe?

YOUR LACTOSE THRESHOLD

The amount of lactose you can ingest without getting symptoms is called your lactose threshold. Each of you has a different threshold, from the equivalent of a few sips of milk to an amount

113

so large you may not exceed it more than once a year. You can't even count on the same amount of lactose producing the same effect each time. Other factors intervene: the type of milk product eaten, its temperature, whether it's eaten alone or with a meal. And don't forget, your threshold is going to drop as you get older and your body produces less and less lactase.

In the meantime, you can easily figure out what your approximate lactose threshold is, close enough so that you know when you've had enough lactose—before the symptoms begin.

Start by drinking a glass of milk. Other milk products will do, but milk is easy to buy, doesn't vary much from one brand to the next, and can easily be taken in large quantities. Begin with an amount you're fairly sure you can handle, say 4 or 8 ounces (½ or 1 cup). Be sure to measure how much you drink, because you should be keeping a careful record of this experiment. Drink the milk by itself, because taking it with different kinds of meals will produce different results. Being consistent is important. Since the idea is to see how much milk you can drink before it affects you, you have to keep other factors as constant as possible. If you drink the milk in the morning the first time, then keep on doing so; don't alternate mornings and evenings. If you wait an hour before eating other foods, always try to keep an hour's gap. The experiment will work best if you tailor it to your daily schedule. Your convenience is important, because you have to be willing to keep trying the same way until you get a result.

One other point before you start: Eating or drinking any additional lactose will throw off all your numbers. So in order to make the experiment work, you must go on a completely lactose-free diet for the entire time you're testing yourself, and even a few days before you begin, to make sure there is no other lactose in your system. Go back and read chapters 5 and 6 if you haven't already done so to learn how to become and stay lactose free. Once you know your lactose threshold, you can go back to your normal diet, as long as you stay under your threshold.

Finally, before you begin, you should lay in a supply of any of the lactase capsules or tablets I describe later in this chapter. Taking the capsules will supply the extra lactase your system lacks and so will relieve or even eliminate the symptoms once you go over your threshold.

Now you're all set. Keep a record of how you feel during the entire test period. Note if you get any symptoms from drinking the milk. Symptoms may include gas, cramps, diarrhea, or a general feeling of discomfort. Your individual symptoms may vary. For some people, symptoms will show up very quickly—within an hour or two. Others may have to wait overnight. If nothing happens, or the symptoms are so mild you're not sure they've been caused by the milk, wait a couple of days for your system to completely get rid of the milk, and try again, with a larger glassful. Keep this up until you start getting obvious or consistent symptoms. (If you get symptoms right away, *decrease* the amount of milk until you *stop* getting symptoms. If any amount at all causes symptoms, then you belong on a lactose-free diet.) That's your threshold. Since milk is about 5 percent lactose, you can then figure out your lactose threshold equivalent (LTE).

The LTE is a device to help you estimate how much of any other milk product you can have without getting symptoms. It tells what the equivalent amount of lactose is in cheese or butter or ice cream or anything else made from milk. As an example, say you started getting symptoms after drinking 10 ounces of milk. I've already said that whole milk is close to 5 percent lactose. If you multiply 10 by 5 percent (or 0.05), you'll see that you were being affected by ½ ounce of lactose. Therefore, you would also be affected by any other food that contained ½ ounce of lactose: 25 ounces of a cheese that is only 2 percent lactose; a mere 4 ounces of sweetened condensed milk. Take a look at the table and chart I've provided for two different ways to determine the proper equivalents for yourself.

(Math buffs rejoice; at last you have a use for that high school algebra. To calculate an LTE: let n equal the number of ounces of milk that cause symptoms. Let y equal the number of ounces of any other milk product you might want to try. Let p equal that product's lactose percentage. You then have an equation that looks like [$y = \frac{0.05n}{p}$] Plug in the numbers—for a person with a lactose threshold of 10 ounces of milk who wants to eat a 2-percent lactose cheese, $n = 10$ and $p = 0.02$—and you get [$y = \frac{0.05 \times 10}{0.02}$]. Therefore $y = 25$.)

My Lactose Threshold Equivalent for Various Foods

FILL IN THE BLANKS.

My lactose threshold is _____ ounces of milk. This is roughly equivalent to:

_____ ounces of butter, Camembert, or Stilton cheese (threshold × 9)

_____ ounces of sherbet, Cheddar, Edam, Gouda, or American cheese (threshold × 2.3)

_____ ounces of American blue, Romadur, or Colby cheese (threshold × 1.8)

_____ ounces of heavy cream, cottage cheese, cream cheese, or Parmesan cheese (threshold × 1.5)

_____ ounces of light whipping cream or sour cream (threshold × 1.3)

_____ ounces of light cream or half-and-half (threshold × 1.1)

_____ ounces of chocolate milk, whole-milk yogurt, or buttermilk (threshold × 1)

_____ ounces of low-fat milk, skim milk, or acidophilus milk (threshold × 0.9)

_____ ounces of yogurt with milk solids added, ice cream, ice milk, or process cheese food (threshold × 0.6)

_____ ounces of evaporated milk (threshold × 0.5)

_____ ounces of sweetened condensed milk (threshold × 0.4)

_____ ounces of whipped cream topping or concentrated milk (threshold × 0.3)

_____ ounces of nonfat dry milk or dry whole milk (threshold × 0.1)

_____ ounces of whey (threshold × 0.07)

LACTOSE THRESHOLD EQUIVALENT FOR AMOUNTS OF FOODS

IF I CAN HAVE THIS MANY OUNCES OF MILK:	THEN I CAN HAVE THIS MANY OUNCES OF A FOOD WHOSE LACTOSE PERCENTAGE IS:									
	1.0	**2.0**	**3.0**	**4.0**	**5.0**	**6.0**	**8.0**	**10.0**	**12.0**	**15.0**
2	10	5	3	3	2	2	1	1	1	1
4	20	10	6	5	4	3	3	2	2	1
6	30	15	10	8	6	5	4	3	3	2
8	40	20	13	10	8	7	5	4	3	3
10	50	25	17	13	10	8	6	5	4	3
12	60	30	20	15	12	10	8	6	5	4
14	70	35	23	18	14	12	9	7	6	5
16	80	40	27	20	16	13	10	8	7	5
18	90	45	30	23	18	15	11	9	8	6
20	100	50	33	25	20	17	13	10	8	7
22	110	55	37	28	22	19	14	11	9	7
24	120	60	40	30	24	20	15	12	10	8

How to use this chart: First determine how many ounces of milk you can drink without getting any symptoms. For example, say the most milk you can drink without getting any symptoms is 12 ounces. This means that in a day's time, you can eat no more lactose from any source than what is contained in 12 ounces of milk. You could have as much as 20 ounces of cottage cheese, which is about 3.0% lactose, or only 8 ounces of vanilla ice milk, which is closer to 8.0% lactose, but not both together. All numbers have been rounded to the nearest ounce. Chapter 5 contains a chart of lactose percentages.

STAYING UNDER YOUR LACTOSE THRESHOLD

By following a few commonsense rules, you can make the most of the room under your lactose threshold, perhaps even have more milk products than your LTE would indicate. As I said before, what you eat and how you eat it has a real effect on your threshold. You can use this fact to your best advantage, a lactose bonus for anyone whose threshold is lower than he or she would like.

1. *Don't overdo it.* The body doesn't keep a store of lactase sitting around just in case some lactose happens to come by. Only when lactose enters the small intestine does lactase production start. By then it can be too late. Those of us with lactose intolerance can only produce so much lactase in a given period of time. That's why it's so easy for the lactose to overwhelm it. The solution is either to cut down on the amount of lactose coming in, so that the threshold is never exceeded, or to spread it out over a longer time, so the body can produce another load of lactase to deal with the lactose.

   Sip a small glass of milk, rather than gulp a large one. Have the pie plain, rather than à la mode. Skip the creamy salad dressing if you have a cream sauce on your meal. Ration the milk products as if they were a special treat you were trying to make last as long as possible (which, in a way, is exactly what they are). Treat the numbers in the Lactose Threshold Equivalent charts as maximums, and stay under them at all times. Remember that lactose is cumulative; every bit of it from every source will contribute toward reaching your threshold. If you forget to check what you eat, or think that each item has so little lactose that it's not even worth considering, you may be surprised by symptoms when you least expect them.

   The great architect Mies van der Rohe once said that less is more. In a way he could never have foreseen, the same is true when it comes to lactose intolerance.

2. *Never drink naked milk.* Lactase has to be in physical contact with lactose in order for it to work. Even if the lactose in a certain food is below your threshold, it may stick around to bother you if it zooms through your intestines so fast that it barely comes in contact with lactase. The speed at which food moves through the digestive tract is called transit time, and for our purposes, slow transit is far better than rapid transit.

   Large meals slow transit time, while a solitary glass of milk moves very quickly. Milk products, therefore, tend to be more digestible if they are consumed with the meal rather than separately. A big dish of ice cream eaten alone late at night will cause more problems than the same dish eaten as dessert.

For the same reason, severely intolerant people are badly affected by the lactose tolerance tests. Taking a large lactose load on an empty stomach places the worst possible stress on someone whose body produces little or no lactose. The resulting symptoms can be painful and lingering.

3. *Eat low-lactose foods*. Whole milk runs about 4.5 to 5.0 percent lactose. Not a high percentage. Yet half of those who are lactose intolerant will develop symptoms after drinking just eight ounces of milk or one-third of an ounce of lactose. If you want to have milk products but are scared off by the lactose percentage in milk, then you need to find products that are as low in lactose as is physically possible. The only two products with lactose percentages lower than 1 percent are butter and ripened cheese.

Foods with high milk fat tend to be lower in lactose than other milk products. Heavy cream is lower in lactose than light cream, which in turn is lower than whole milk. Butter is higher in fat than any of these, and in turn is the lowest in lactose. Estimates vary considerably, but the highest figure I've seen for butter's lactose content is 1 percent; the lowest is a bare .06 percent.

You would think that butter would be the one milk product that would be acceptable for mildly lactose-intolerant individuals. Authorities disagree. Some doctors, and the authors of every lactose-reduced diet I've ever seen, insist that butter not be included in the diet. Butter's high fat content is cited as an additional reason to avoid it. Many people, it seems, have trouble digesting fats. This may be related to the potential for milk-fat intolerance I mention in Chapter 4, or it may simply be that fats in and of themselves can cause stomach distress for certain people. My recommendation for butter has to be one of cautious experimentation. But, unless you have very severe lactose intolerance, you may not have to give butter up at all.

The other low-lactose milk product is less risky to recommend. As cheese ripens, the bacteria in it ferment lactose to lactic acid, giving certain cheeses their characteristic sharp tang and lowering the lactose content, possibly to zero. Few fats are left, either; ripened cheeses are mostly protein. Usually the more aged the cheese, the lower its lactose content. Camembert, Stilton, aged Cheddar, and aged Swiss are all common cheeses with low lactose contents.

4. *A dose of culture is good for you.* Bacteria find their way into milk products other than cheeses. Sour creams, buttermilk, acidophilus milk, and yogurt are also cultured with bacteria. Since the role of the bacteria is to convert the lactose into lactic acid, in theory, cultured milk products should be low in lactose and therefore safe to eat or drink.

Half that statement is correct. People with lactose intolerance do seem to tolerate cultured milk products better than straight milk. But not because the products are low in lactose. Yogurt, in fact, can have a higher lactose percentage than whole milk.

Yogurt is made by adding milk solids—usually nonfat dry milk—to bulk up whole or skim milk by 30 percent. This produces a food that well deserves the name health food, being 30 percent higher in protein and calcium than milk by itself. It is also, however, 30 percent higher in lactose. Two strains of bacteria—*Streptococcus thermophilus* and *Lactobacillus bulgaricus*—are added to ferment the high-nutrient milk mixture and turn it into yogurt. About 30 percent of the lactose is broken down in this process—only enough to bring yogurt's lactose percentage back down to that of milk.

The secret of yogurt's digestibility lies in the bacteria themselves. The bacterial cultures survive the trip down your digestive tract and are still active when they reach your large intestine. Once there, they while away the time busily manufacturing lactase—enough lactase to digest the lactose they brought along with them. In other words, yogurt digests itself, whether or not you have lactase in your system.

This theory may need revision, but there is no doubt that yogurt is the best-tolerated milk product, capable of being eaten even by people with severe lactose intolerance (although some people do suffer some of the familiar symptoms of lactose intolerance after eating yogurt).

Plain yogurt also makes an excellent substitute for sour cream. Yogurt separates during cooking, however. To prevent this, mix one tablespoon of cornstarch with one tablespoon of yogurt, and then stir the mixture into one cup of yogurt. Stir over medium heat until thickened.

5. *Be a chocaholic*. Drink chocolate milk. Sure, chocolate milk is frowned upon by the food purists. Yes, chocolate inhibits calcium absorption, so you defeat one of the major purposes of drinking milk by adding chocolate to it. No, nobody is quite sure why chocolate milk is better tolerated than unflavored milk. (One theory is that it moves through the digestive tract more slowly, thereby giving whatever lactase your system produces a better chance at the lactose.) Have fun. Be a kid again.

6. *Read food labels*. The day the government required food processors to list ingredients on the labels of their products should be called National Lactose Intolerance Liberation Day. Reading the ingredients list on every single product purchased is the smartest thing anyone with lactose intolerance can do. Not only can you tell when a product is completely milk free, but you should also be able to take a good guess at which products are so low in lactose that they might be safe for the mildly intolerant.

Any ingredient used in amounts as small as half an ounce will probably be well down the list, and seemingly insignificant. Yet half an ounce of dried whey contains as much lactose as eight ounces of whole milk. Other whey products and most dried milk products have lactose percentages in the double digits. Avoiding foods with any mention of these products is a good rule. Staying away from foods with more than one milk product listed is also good advice.

Lactose percentages in milk products have already been discussed at greater length in Chapter 5.

7. *Eat lactose-reduced foods*. Milk-free foods and milk substitutes have been around for a long time. The idea of lactose-reduced products is a new one, dating only from the early 1980s, when manufacturers finally realized that there was a market large enough to be worth making an effort to serve it.

If you shop around, at least on the East Coast, you should be able to find lactose-reduced brands of milk, ice cream, cottage cheese, and pasteurized process cheese food. All these products have about 70 percent of the normal amount of lactose removed. For milk, this means having around 1.5 percent

lactose instead of the normal 5.0 percent. In other words, if
you could have 10 ounces of regular milk, you could have 33
ounces of the lactose-reduced milk.

The major supplier of lactose-reduced products is Lactaid,
Inc., which I talk about in the following sections. Lactaid
distributes its milk through local dairies or milk cooperatives.
Giving Lactaid milk its first competition is Enjoy Lactose
Reduced Lowfat Milk, marketed through the giant Kroger supermarket chain. Enjoy milk also starts out 70 percent lactose
free, but because it does not go through Lactaid's ultrapas-
teurization process, the lactase enzyme continues to stay active, digesting even more lactose. The milk never becomes
completely lactose free, however. It's currently being marketed
mainly in the midwest. A whole line of other low-lactose
products are in the planning stages. Friendship Foods also
supplies a Lactose Reduced Lowfat Cottage Cheese. Check
your local supermarkets to see if these or similar products are
carried or can be ordered.

LACTASE IN A PILL . . . AND MORE

The greatest breakthrough in products for the lactose intolerant
has been the development of pills and liquids that provide the
lactase enzyme that we lack. These come in two forms, one that
gets added to milk or other liquids and that actually breaks down
the lactose before you drink it, and one that is swallowed as a
tablet or capsule whenever you're having a solid food containing
lactose.

I've included the lactase products here in the chapter on a
lactose-reduced diet because none of them does a perfect job of
removing lactose. It is difficult if not impossible to judge accu-
rately how many pills to take to balance the uncertain amount of
lactose in your food. Some people find that the lactose can linger
in their systems longer than the effects of the pill. Taking more
pills help, but the balancing act is always uncertain. Still, the
success rate of these products is remarkable, and even people
with severe lactose intolerance, like myself, find that they can

have an occasional milk product with no or few ill effects. For traveling, special dinners, or any time when the choice may be eating food with some lactose or not eating at all, they are absolutely essential.

The two major names in the market are Lactaid and Lactrase. I'll take up each separately, and also mention several other, smaller firms that market similar products.

A warning: All these lactase-containing products work by splitting the lactose in foods into the simpler sugars glucose and galactose. If you are diabetic, you need to consult your doctor to see how this additional sugar will affect you. If you have galactosemia, then you should not use any of these products at all, as the release of galactose could be dangerous.

THE EVER-GROWING LACTAID FAMILY

A few of you with long memories may still nostalgically recall the day nearly ten years ago when your local health food store received its first shipment of a fantastic new product, a powder that would actually make milk safe to drink. Unlike some of the claims that occasionally get bandied around health food stores, this one was indeed true. And if the contortions necessary to get the product to work resembled the wilder flights of a medieval alchemist, that was a small price to pay for the comforting splash of cold milk on cereal first thing in the morning.

Today's product, still cleverly named Lactaid and still manufactured by Lactaid, Inc., a subsidiary of the SugarLo Company, is more sophisticated, easier to use, and just one of a family of wares aimed at the lactose intolerant. (As an aside, the product was originally spelled Lact-Aid, which was changed to LactAid, and is being converted to today's Lactaid. Mysterious are the ways of marketers.)

The idea behind Lactaid is a simple one. We know that a variety of one-celled creatures have the ability to manufacture the lactase enzyme, since we have colonies of bacteria in our intestines that can do exactly that. Why not, then, feed lactose to specially grown yeast (*Kluyveromyces lactis*, if you care) and collect the lactase they produce? Making lactase this way qualifies it as a food and not a drug under federal rules.

Lactaid today mixes the lactase enzyme with a liquid consisting of 50 percent glycerol, 30 percent water, and 20 percent inert yeast dry matter. Unlike the original powder, this liquid mixes quickly and easily with most types of milk—whole, skim, low fat, reconstituted, chocolate, and canned. You can even use it on cottage cheese, puddings, or ice cream. It shouldn't be added directly to buttermilk or other cultured milk products (including yogurt) because of their high acid content.

Lactaid comes in little applicator bottles in 1-, 3-, 7-, and 19-milliliter sizes. The Lactaid people call these 4-, 12-, 30-, and 75-quart sizes, but this is very approximate because each person may need to use different amounts of Lactaid in milk.

Here's how it works: Assume you're treating a quart of fresh milk (it has to be fresh; Lactaid won't work if the milk is too old). Squeeze 4 to 5 drops of Lactaid into the milk carton. Shake *very well*. Store the milk in the refrigerator for twenty-four hours. This will remove 70 percent of the lactose in the milk, converting it to glucose and galactose in the same way your body would if it manufactured lactase.

People who are more severely lactose intolerant can't, of course, take even 30 percent lactose. More Lactaid helps this problem. A double dose, 8 to 10 drops, removes more than 90 percent of the lactose. A triple dose, 12 to 15 drops, gets rid of 99-plus percent of the lactose. Using 8 to 10 drops, but waiting forty-eight hours, should have the same effect. No dosage will ever make milk 100-percent-guaranteed lactose free, but this should come very close.

After letting the milk sit for the twenty-four hours, use it exactly as you would any other milk—for drinking, in cooking, in cereals—any way you want. It will taste slightly sweeter than untreated milks, because glucose and galactose are sweeter than lactose, but it will look and act otherwise the same.

Lactaid should be used in other liquid milk products (cream, for example) in the same dosage: 4 to 5 drops per quart for a normal dose, double or triple that for greater lactose breakdown.

Yes, some of the liquid milk products contain less lactose than whole milk, but their higher fat content makes it harder for the enzyme to work efficiently, so the two factors cancel each other out. At least you don't have to remember a new set of numbers every time you add Lactaid.

A bit of common sense is needed whenever you use Lactaid. Don't assume that the 70-percent level is sufficient and then find out you're wrong by drinking a quart of milk for the first time in two years. Go slow. Use a double dose the first time out, and only have a small amount of whatever you're testing it in. If no symptoms develop, then reduce the dose or eat or drink more. Experiment until you figure out what works best for you. You should have plenty of time. You can use Lactaid up to two years after you buy it.

No Lack of Lactaid

Once all of America could buy Lactaid, in supermarkets and drugstores as well as health food stores, the company went searching for new worlds to conquer. Competition from other products forced them to ask the big question: Why should people have to wait twenty-four or more hours to drink their milk? The company couldn't speed up the enzyme, so they did the next best thing. Lactaid is now marketing a whole line of lactose-reduced products right in your neighborhood supermarket dairy case.

Their hot new product is Lactaid Specially Digestible Lactose Reduced Milk, mixed so that 70 percent of the lactose is removed. The milk only comes in a low fat (1 percent milk fat) variety, so those who want lactose-reduced whole milk will still have to make it at home. Lactaid liquid can be added to the reduced lactose milk, if you need to reduce the lactose even further. Use about 8 drops, even though the amount of lactose is low, for best results. Supermarkets in most areas (maybe two-thirds) of the country should have the milk available.

Other Lactaid products were just beginning to be introduced as this chapter was being written, so it may be awhile before you see them in your stores. Lactaid Specially Digestible Cottage Cheese is getting regional distribution in the Northeast. Lactaid Specially Digestible American Pasteurized Process Cheese Food will hit New England, Philadelphia, Florida, and then California. Lactaid Specially Digestible Ice Cream—in four flavors: vanilla, chocolate, raspberry swirl, and vanilla fudge—is available along the East Coast. All have 70 percent of their lactose removed.

Beyond Milk

Because of the form of lactase produced by the yeast used to make Lactaid, it shouldn't be used directly on hot or acidic foods. (Hot foods include cocoa, creamed soups, or cheese pizza. Acidic foods include most creamy salad dressings, sour cream, yogurt, and other cultured milk products.) The Lactaid people recommend that you mix the Lactaid with a spoonful of milk first and then just eat those foods straight. Of course, milk that has already been treated with Lactaid can later be heated or turned into yogurt.

The body is another highly acidic environment, and Lactaid simply isn't as efficient working there as it is in milk. The mixing-Lactaid-with-milk bit is also clumsy enough that I doubt many people bother. For the times when you would like to eat hot or acidic foods, or just when you want a solid food containing lactose, having a handy pill to take would be a whole lot simpler. Other companies saw this first, and Lactaid followed their lead in early 1985.

Lactaid tablets contain a slightly different form of the lactase enzyme, which is better suited for use in a person's digestive system. Again, experimentation is needed to determine the proper dosage for each person, which will also vary depending upon what it is you're eating. Fortunately, the package explicitly says, "Absolutely safe at any level of use." The filler in the tablet is dicalcium phosphate, which is very unlikely to cause a reaction of its own.

Each tablet contains at least 3300 FDA lactase units. All other manufacturers of lactase tablets provide measurement of strength in milligrams. The Lactaid people claim that the two measurement units are not strictly comparable but admit that Lactaid tablets contain 111 milligrams of lactase.

FOR MORE INFO, CALL . . .

If you can't find a local store that carries the Lactaid liquid or tablets, you can have your pharmacist call the Lactaid toll-free number, 800-257-8650 (in New Jersey it's 609-645-7500, which is not free), to place an order. You can use the hot line yourself between 8:30 and 4:00 Eastern time if you have questions about any of the products or their uses. However, Lactaid liquid and tablets can be found most everywhere in the United States and Canada, in Guatemala, and overseas in Israel, the Middle East, and Australia.

LACTASE IN A CAPSULE

Okay, there's Lactaid liquid and Lactaid tablets, so Lactaid must have the market cornered, right? Not by a long shot. There's one other way of using lactase that has a number of advantages all its own. Here the big name is Lactrase, made by the Kremens-Urban Company.

Lactrase comes in a capsule, which, for many people, makes it easier to swallow than a tablet. Each capsule contains 125 milligrams of lactase, more than in any other lactase-containing product I'm aware of. One Lactrase capsule is designed to digest approximately half the lactose in an eight-ounce glass of milk. If you're more lactose intolerant than the norm, simply take more Lactrase capsules until you stop having symptoms. Always start high and experiment until you find the right dosage for yourself. Fortunately, if you guess wrong and start too low, all you need do is take more Lactrase when the symptoms start; it will work as long as there is lactose in your system.

If that's all it did, Lactrase would still be a great boon to the lactose intolerant. But the clever people at Kremens-Urban made the capsules openable—and that opens up a whole range of possibilities.

Relief Is Just a Swallow Away

You want the lactase to be in contact with the lactose for as long as possible. Swallowing a capsule may interfere with that, as some people's digestive juices don't dissolve capsules very well. Solving that problem takes only a second—just long enough to open the capsule.

Pouring the white Lactrase powder directly on whatever you plan to eat makes it more effective, ensuring that it begins to work as soon as you swallow it. Every extra minute means that much more lactose that is broken down and made harmless. Sprinkling the Lactrase on foods doesn't change the taste—unless you get too much of it in one spot, in which case the effect is a little like eating cornstarch, mostly because the filler Lactrase uses in its capsule is malto-dextrin, also derived from corn.

Everything you can do to keep the Lactrase in touch with the lactose makes it work that much better. If you are having a meal with several sources of lactose—say, a creamy salad dressing, followed by fish sautéed in butter, with cake and ice cream for dessert—you may need to take several pills. Don't worry, Lactrase is safe and effective even at high doses. Taking the extra capsules with or pouring them on each lactose source ensures longer contact and makes you less likely to develop symptoms. If you guess wrong about how much lactose is in a meal—easy to do—more Lactrase taken that night or the next day, whenever the symptoms begin, will help you feel better.

One small problem with the malto-dextrin is that it doesn't dissolve well in liquids. It works, but it leaves little lumps behind, making it even tougher to face your morning coffee than usual. Swallow a pill with the coffee instead.

Both Lactrase and the Lactaid tablets derive their lactase from the same source, *Aspergillus oryzae*, which is a different fungus than the one used for Lactaid liquid. This is necessary in order to get a variety of lactase that will work in an acidic environment like the stomach. Because Lactrase has a specialized function, it is not quite as efficient if poured into milk. If one capsule removes 50 percent of the lactose in 8 ounces of milk if swallowed, it will only remove 35 percent if poured into milk and left in the refrigerator a day to sit. Using one extra capsule per 8 ounces of milk will make the effect equal, however.

THERE'LL BE A HOT LINE IN THE OLD TOWN TONIGHT

Lactrase capsules come in bottles of 100 pills. They're nonprescription but are sometimes only available from behind the pharmacist's counter rather than on drugstore or supermarket shelves. This is so the pharmacist can break open a bottle and give you a smaller quantity of the pills if you choose. If your pharmacist doesn't carry them, he or she can get them within forty-eight hours from the Rorer wholesaler. (Rorer is the parent company of Kremens-Urban.) Lactrase capsules are not available outside the United States.

If you would like more information, there is of course a toll-free number to call: 800-558-5114.

OTHER LACTASE SOURCES

I don't want to give you the impression that Lactaid and Lactrase are the only products out there that will help you drink milk again. They're just the biggest names and so probably the easiest to find. I know of four other sources for lactase, and there are undoubtedly many more in health food stores across the nation.

LACTOZYME

Lactozyme is very much like the early powder version of Lactaid. It's designed to be added to milk—whole, skim, reconstituted from powder, whey, condensed, or canned—and will remove about 75 percent of the lactose in twenty-four hours. It comes in capsule form but is *not* supposed to be swallowed. Write to Schiff Bio-Food Products, Moonachie NJ 07074.

SUPER MILK DIGESTANT

Malabar Formulas makes Super Milk Digestant tablets. Each pill contains 50 milligrams of lactase and also contains 4 milligrams of rennin. The rennin is there because it's useful for curdling the milk protein, casein, which makes the digested food more acceptable to the lactase, predigesting it, in a way.

The lactase in Super Milk Digestant also comes from our old friend *Aspergillus oryzae*. Just to confuse you further, it contains 5000 Ortho Nitro Phenol Galactoside units per gram, which is equal to 166.7 FDA units. The government has yet to establish a standard way of measuring the effectiveness of an enzyme.

One tablet of Super Milk Digestant should aid in the digestion of 4 ounces of milk, buttermilk, or kefir (a type of fermented milk), 5 ounces of yogurt, or 8 ounces of cottage cheese, according to the manufacturer. Of course, you will still need to experiment to determine the proper dosage for yourself.

Shelf life is approximately two years under normal storage conditions. To make them last that long, keep the tablets in a cool (below 85° F), dry, dark area, away from direct sunlight.

Super Milk Digestant is available in 50-, 100-, 150-, and 250-tablet sizes from health- and natural-food stores throughout the United States and in Canada, England, and Australia. For more information, write to Malabar Formulas, 28537 Neuvo Valley Drive, P.O. Box 3, Neuvo, CA 92367, or call 714-657-3438.

Milk Gest

Milk Gest, from Nu-Life, also is a lactase-rennin combination, with 25 milligrams of lactase and 4 milligrams of rennin per tablet. Available in health- and natural-food stores, it's manufactured for Gides-Nulife, Incorporated, Orange CA 92667.

Milk Digestant

Natural Blend Milk Digestant Tablets are a third variety of lactase-rennin tablets. These have 25 milligrams of lactase and 2 milligrams of rennin. They are available only by mail or at GNC natural food stores, and are distributed by Natural Sales Company, Pittsburgh, PA 15230.

A PRICE COMPARISON

Lactase-containing tablets and capsules come in different strengths, with different added ingredients, and contain different amounts of lactase, all of which makes price comparisons in the store very difficult. After all, a $4.49 bottle of Milk Gest looks much cheaper than a $27.98 bottle of Lactrase. Looks are deceiving. I've tried to standardize the variants somewhat by, where possible, looking only at bottles containing 100 tablets or capsules (larger size bottles are almost always cheaper per pill than the smaller bottles) and then adjusting for the amount of lactase. Here's what the various pills cost me, per 100 milligrams of lactase.

Lactrase	$0.22
Lactaid	$0.17
Super Milk Digestant	$0.18
Milk Gest	$0.18
Milk Digestant	$0.12*

*Price for 250 tablet bottle.

The difference in price per dose is really rather small. Rather than deciding by price, I'd recommend you let individual effectiveness, availability, convenience, and versatility determine which of the products you use.

CHAPTER EIGHT
LACTOSE IN THE SUPERMARKET

The days of the homemaker mother creating meals for a hungry brood from scratch are long gone, if they ever existed outside the golden haze of a middle-class media. Americans today eat packaged food purchased at American supermarkets. Even those of you who buy fresh vegetables and meat at the farm market, butcher shop, or health food store usually manage to accumulate a bevy of packaged, canned, frozen, bottled, or otherwise processed foods in your kitchen cabinets.

Kick and scream all you will; sooner or later, you'll have to go into the supermarket and start to apply all that knowledge about food you've picked up in the last three chapters.

I wish I could just give you a list of foods and say, avoid these, they contain lactose. It can't be done. Just about any food you can think of is made by somebody, somewhere, with milk products. At the same time, you can almost always find either a substitute or a milk-free version of what you need to complete a recipe.

You're best off learning what you can and cannot have the hard way—by reading the ingredients list on the label of every single product you lay your hands on. Doing so gives you the crucial experience to know what's available that suits your own idiosyncratic tastes. Besides, products and product lines vary enormously from one part of the country to another, and advice that works in one region doesn't always work a few hundred miles away. Some companies even adapt their recipes to differing regional tastes, so that a product that is milk-free in the Northeast may contain milk in the Southwest.

Given all that, here are a few general tips on what to expect in the supermarket, from someone who's spent hours walking up and down aisles, reading the ingredients lists on every product. I start with the word that guarantees lactose-free safety to everyone with lactose intolerance—*pareve*.

Pareve: When Kosher Ain't Kosher Enough

Most people have heard of kosher food—food prepared according to the Jewish dietary laws. If you have, then you probably know that (along with a million other things) mixing milk and meat is strictly forbidden. Obeying the law requires a scrupulous conscientiousness that affects every aspect of food preparation.

Before the advent of food labeling laws, it was next to impossible to tell exactly what was in commercially prepared foods. Manufacturers responded to the very real need of Jewish families to know what was in the foods on store shelves by preparing— and boldly labeling—foods that could be eaten with either milk meals or meat meals: neutral foods. (This occurred only because the food industry saw that there existed a large, cohesive, and highly motivated market for such products—a lesson for the lactose intolerant.)

These foods are called *pareve* (sometimes spelled *parve*), variously pronounced in the real world to rhyme with *carve* or *Harvey*. If you believe the dictionary, however, it's pronounced *PAH-ruh-vuh*. No matter. You probably will never have to say it if you just remember that the word *pareve* on the side of a food package label means that the food is completely and guaranteedly milk free.

Some people (even nutrition textbooks!) make the mistake of assuming that anything kosher is safe for the lactose intolerant. Wrong, and potentially dangerous. Not all kosher foods are pareve and not all pareve foods are kosher. Any dairy product prepared under the guidance of a specially trained rabbi can be marked kosher, but that doesn't help us any. Similarly, a great many everyday supermarket brands aren't in the least bit kosher but are thoroughly and completely pareve. All kosher products containing any meat, however, must of necessity also be milk free.

This also might help explain the puzzling references to "vegetarian" in foods like Campbell's Vegetarian Vegetable Soup or Heinz Vegetarian Beans, ordinary supermarket products that seem to have no connection to a specialty market. Most regular vegetable soups use a stock made from beef, which would disqualify the soup from being pareve. The word *vegetarian* in the name indicates that nothing from an animal has been used in its preparation. A vegetable soup made with beef stock could be lactose-free without being pareve. It's a tricky business.

Another source of confusion is the designation "kosher-style." True kosherness, with all its rules and regulations, is an expensive proposition. Many manufacturers try to get the look and appeal of kosher foods (especially delicatessen foods) without the fuss and bother. To a few, any hot dog they leave the pork out of is "kosher-style." More reputable operators make a far greater effort to make their foods very close to kosher, so they refuse to add fillers such as milk products to their meats. You can probably rely upon most delis serving "kosher-style" food or companies selling "kosher-style" products, such as breads, to be as good bets for the lactose intolerant as kosher would be. Just be careful that the "kosher-style" deli doesn't serve you sour cream on your baked potato.

Real kosher foods are hard to find, except in stores in cities with sizable Jewish populations. If you can find a Jewish bakery nearby, you may be in for a real treat. Most breads in a Jewish bakery—rye, pumpernickel, chollah, and bagels and rolls—are pareve. In some bakeries, many of the goodies are also baked without milk. I've even found milk-free pumpkin pies. (Delicious, I might add.) Sometimes the bakery will bake pareve cakes and cookies to order, if given advance notice. Kosher delis are also good places to get thoroughly acquainted with. It's no accident that kosher corned beef on real New York Jewish rye bread is world-famous.

Pareve foods may be found over most of the country because of the national firms that have placed the word on their labels. Pareve is not a cure-all for the trials of lactose-free shopping, but in the absence of large "lactose-free" labels plastered all over food packages, it's the best thing we've got.

WHERE LACTOSE LURKS

Once you are past the guarantee represented by foods marked *pareve*, you're on your own in a supermarket. Manufacturers sometimes hide lactose in very unlikely places, while in other foods, you have to hunt through a whole section to find one that doesn't contain lactose. Recipes often change, too, so you need to check the ingredients lists every time you go to the store, even if it's a product you've been using for years. Recently I discovered that a brand of whole wheat bread I had long relied on suddenly listed whey among the ingredients. I didn't follow my own rules: I was home, with a bite of bread actually in my mouth, before I bothered to read the list.

What follows is a generalist's guide to the grocery store. Use it to get yourself familiar with the tricky ins and outs of lactose-free shopping. By the way, when I say that a food is safe or okay, I mean only that it is lactose-free. You will still need to check foods for other products to which you may be allergic or sensitive. And, of course, any specific brand name product I mention may change its ingredients at any time, so be sure to double-check the ingredients for yourself when you go shopping.

BEVERAGES

Instant coffees appear in the "Avoid" columns of several of the lactose-free diets I looked at while researching this book, but I have yet to find an example of any coffee, either regular or decaffeinated, that contains lactose. (Some people have a sensitivity to caffeine, which produces symptoms very similar to those of lactose intolerance. As far as I am aware, there is no connection between the two, however.) Postum grain beverages are also lactose free. Even the various international coffee lines with added ingredients to make them "Swiss" or "Irish" are safe, although the ones from General Mills contain sodium caseinate.

Hot chocolates are less trustworthy. Pure cocoa is safe to drink (if not made with added milk), and so are the Quiks, chocolate and strawberry; but virtually everything else on the shelves is betrayed by the name "cocoa mix." Cocoa mixes all come ready-made with sugar and some form of milk. Make your own hot chocolate directly from cocoa; it tastes just as good and will have less sugar.

Teas, both traditional and herbal, are lactose free.

Kool-Aid is another product some people have accused of containing lactose, but its maker, General Foods, places every flavor in all three types—unsweetened, sugar-sweetened, and sugar-free—on its lactose-free list.

Fruit juices of all kinds are possibly the best substitute for milk, and you can even bake with them. Beware the difference between fruit juices and fruit drinks. The latter are cheaper but contain much less real fruit juice and much more added sugar. Both, however, are lactose free.

Say what you want about the calories, artificial sweeteners, phosphoric acids, and gas-producing carbonation of soft drinks; at least they don't contain lactose—with the exception, that is, of Yoo Hoo Chocolate, Strawberry, and Coconut Flavored Drinks, whose ingredients include milk and whey. (Yoo Hoo Diet Chocolate Fudge Artificially Flavored Soda is okay, however, presumably because it's impossible to take all the calories out of a food and leave any milk products in.)

Covering all the alcoholic beverages in the world would take another book. As a quick guide, beers and wines are okay, but beware of the cream added to many fashionable liquors and drinks.

BREADS AND ROLLS

Breads can be summarized by one simple rule: The closer the bread is to ordinary commercial white bread, the more likely it is to have lactose. Virtually all white breads have whey or nonfat dry milk added to them. So do many of the soft, pale wheat and rye breads made by the big commercial bakers. And so do most of the big fluffy dinner, hot dog, and sandwich rolls as well. English muffins, like other rolls, are usually made with milk, but at least the ones that pretend to be health foods, made from whole wheat or with added raisins or suchlike, can sometimes be found milk free.

The safest breads are the ones made with the fewest ingredients. Most true French and Italian breads are quite safe. Breads that pretend to be true Jewish-style rye or pumpernickel will ordinarily be made without any milk products. Pareve breads, of course, are totally safe. Heavy whole wheat breads, especially the ones made without preservatives by small natural foods bakeries, are also good bets, though a few contain milk because it is, after all, such a good source of nutrients.

If you want an everyday white bread that is safe, you'll have to go out and search for it. Certain companies make a "European" bread American-style: that is, a French, Italian, or Vienna bread that is baked, sliced, and packaged to look like regular white bread. I've used them for many years, and they make fine sandwich breads, without the spongy texture of a whipped American white bread.

Bread mixes have become one of the latest prepared food fads, specially developed to take most of the work out of kneading and working the dough for long periods of time. If you don't try to get too exotic, you may find some to be safe. Muffin mixes, on the other hand, abound in milk-free varieties. For a change, experiment with a good old-fashioned cornbread mix, most brands of which are okay.

Finding a commercial source of milk-free bread crumbs is a project for a fifty-person scavenger hunt. Every time I think I've finally latched onto a reliable brand, it disappears from the shelves. If you can't find a Jewish bakery, make your own bread crumbs. Either of two methods will work: Let the bread you normally use turn dry and stale, and then crumble (true crumbs can only come from crumbling); or simply toss either fresh or stale bread briefly into a blender.

Over in the refrigerator case lie ready-to-heat rolls and muffins in those weird cardboard tubes you open by pushing in with a spoon until the dough explodes all over your kitchen. Don't get scared off by all the labels proclaiming *buttermilk* in large letters. The smaller print often says "artificially flavored," and by careful reading of ingredient lists, you can make in minutes hot, flaky, buttery rolls to fool your friends, provided you don't let them in on the secret that you're spreading milk-free margarine on top.

Cake Mixes and Cookie Mixes

Surprise! The vast majority of cake mixes on supermarket shelves have no milk products in them. Not all, certainly—pudding-mix cakes almost always have some milk, as do cakes with fillings—but hordes of chocolate, yellow, and variety cakes made by such big names as Duncan Hines, Betty Crocker, and Pillsbury are perfectly safe. Since they usually only call for adding oil, eggs, and water, you don't even have to come up with a milk-free margarine.

I've always made my own frostings (for cooked frostings, substitute Coffee Rich for the milk; for "buttercream" frostings, use milk-free margarine in place of the butter), but some of you no doubt appreciate the convenience of the commercial ready-to-spread varieties. Trying to find the pattern that will let you predict which frostings will be safe will keep you up nights. Duncan Hines, for example, uses nonfat milk in its Vanilla Frosting but not in Chocolate Creamy; more nonfat milk in Milk Chocolate but not in Double Dutch Fudge. Keep trying brands until you find the frosting you need.

Far fewer cookie mixes appear on store shelves than do cake mixes (I wonder why?), and only a handful are milk free. As with the frostings, however, some searching should provide you a fair amount of variety among the different brands.

Pies are a problem. First off, most pie crusts sold commercially use milk products. In addition, custard and cream pies are automatically out. If you insist on buying a pie, look for a fruit pie on a milk-free crust, but you might be better off learning to bake.

CEREALS

For most cereals, the only question you have to ask is, what in the world can I put on them when I can't have milk? If you're only mildly lactose intolerant, I'd suggest trying a reduced-lactose milk, either one bought commercially or made at home with the use of Lactaid or a similar product (see Chapter 7).

In the world of substitutions, you could try diluting Coffee Rich with water to bring it to the consistency of milk. Soy milks are another way of approximating the flavor and texture of milk. Some people pour juices on their cereal, Hawkeye Pierce on *M*A*S*H* used beer, and several hot cereals can be made with water in place of the milk.

Until I went to the store and looked, it never occurred to me that the cereals themselves would contain milk products, but some do. They range from such "adult" varieties as Total, Special K, and Quaker 100% Natural, to kiddie favorites like Cap'n Crunch's Crunchberries, all of which contain either nonfat dry milk or whey. (Post uses milk protein in its Fortified Oat Flakes and S'Mores Crunch.) A few of the more exotic flavors among the instant hot cereals also contain milk products. Although the number of problem-causing cereals is probably no more than a dozen, that should be enough to keep you on your toes when you enter the cereal aisle.

COOKIES AND CRACKERS

Chocolate lovers of the world—learn to bake. In my younger days, there were only two kinds of cookies in the world, chocolate and chocolate chip. I still head for them when I go to the supermarket today, but to my disappointment as I wander up and down the cookie aisle, virtually everything with chocolate in it also contains milk. Not all. For some incomprehensible reason, I know of brands whose chocolate chocolate chip cookies are milk free but whose chocolate chips are not. Go figure.

When you grow tired of the one or two kinds of chocolate cookies that are safe, you may find yourself growing to like a whole range of other cookies that are much easier to find milk free. Vanilla, oatmeal, molasses, and ginger cookies—all the old-fashioned kind—might get you through a junk food seizure until you can find a handy recipe and bake your own.

Crackers are more straightforward, since your basic saltine cracker is easily available milk free. A wide variety of other crackers also turn out to be safe, ranging from the dry toasted rye or sesame crackers to Ritz Crackers to more exotic party crackers. Several brands of graham crackers make the safe list as well, a terrific plus for baking, since graham cracker crusts (made with milk-free margarine, of course) form the bases for any number of tasty pies. Several ready-made graham cracker and regular pie crusts also exist milk free, another aid for us fumble-fingered would-be bakers.

Fruits and Vegetables

Have as much and as many as you want of fresh fruits and vegetables. Once they're packaged, however, strange things can happen.

A surprising number of lactose-free diets warn people to stay away from frozen or fast-food french fries. French fries, depending upon moisture content, cooking time, and fat temperature, don't always develop that golden brown glow that we've been brought up to believe is the proper color for the perfect fry. Where nature fails, science provides. A sugar coating sprayed onto the potato slice turns it a beautiful shade of brown during the frying.

If that sugar coating were to be lactose, then we'd have a problem. But all the french fries I've been able to check, including those of frozen food giant Ore-Ida and the universally top-rated fast food fries at McDonald's, are sprayed with a different sugar— dextrose—instead. Somebody must have been spraying their french fries with lactose at one time, though, so don't take those ingredients labels for granted. Regardless, long before I'd worry about the faint chance of fries containing lactose, I'd find many another thing to worry about.

Butter sauces, for one. Cream sauces, for another. The new

emphasis on more healthful meals has led frozen-food manufacturers to develop scores of delicious-looking vegetables and vegetable combinations, all drowning in butter and cream sauces.
As if those weren't bad enough, another whole section of the
frozen vegetable bin is filled with packages topped off with cheese
sauce. Stay away from anything marked "au gratin," for it's sure
to have cheese inside.

The hottest new food of all, led by Stouffer's astoundingly
successful Lean Cuisine, is the low-calorie high-priced gourmet
frozen entrée including meats and vegetables. No gourmet would
ever think of cooking vegetables in anything other than butter,
and Stouffer's and all its imitators follow suit. Green Giant makes
a bare handful of entrées that are safe, but for the most part, you
should avoid the twenty feet of freezer case these yuppie children
of the lowly TV dinner have taken over for their own. For that
matter, avoid TV dinners as well.

Fortunately, most vegetables and many fruits are available either frozen or canned without the added sauces that can give us
so much trouble. Canned vegetables, as a group, are more likely
than frozen vegetables over all to be lactose-free. The only exceptions I can come up with off the top of my head are B in B
brand canned mushrooms. B in B stands for Broiled in Butter.

Some lactose-free diets recommend staying away from canned
peas because of added lactose. This advice is as good as the
advice about french fries. I have not come across any manufacturer who adds lactose to peas. Sure, almost every can of peas
lists sugar among its ingredients, but the Food and Drug Administration says that sugar on a label means sucrose, not lactose.
The FDA also allows manufacturers to add butter or margarine
to canned peas, as well as virtually every other canned vegetable,
but the manufacturer has to say so on the ingredients list. Check
and be sure, by all means, but don't stay away from canned peas
just out of suspicion.

Several firms have varieties of instant potatoes that are lactose
free. Coffee Rich and milk-free margarine need to be added. I
haven't tried soy milk in instant mashed potatoes, but I see no
reason it wouldn't work. Just try not to serve them to any health
food purists among your acquaintances.

Salad Dressings

Commercial salad dressings are, from our point of view, fortunate fakes. Over and over again, you'll notice the front label on the bottle proclaiming "Creamy" French or "Creamy" Italian, only to find, to your relief, that absolutely nothing in the bottle remotely resembles cream.

Many "creamy" dressings are really mayonnaise based, which means that they can be eaten in perfect safety by the lactose intolerant. Most of the store-bought Russian and Thousand Island dressings fall into this category as well. French dressings are my dressing of choice in restaurants because they very seldom contain any milk products. Of course, oil-and-vinegar and clear Italian dressings are good alternatives if no French is available, if you have your doubts about its milk-free standing, or if you just prefer them.

Just when you thought it was safe to browse through the dressings, the latest fad among the manufacturers is buttermilk and cream cheese dressings, all of which use depressingly real milk products. Too bad, for these offer a range of choices among dressings with no real equivalents among the milk-free varieties.

Soups

You may think that all you have to do is avoid the various cream of ... soups, but life is much more complicated than that. Take a simple pea soup, for example. Lipton's Cup-a-Soup contains some milk products, but Progresso, Grandma Brown's, and Stouffer's frozen pea soup don't. Stick to a single company, then? Take Campbell's. Their condensed Green Pea has lactose in it but their Chunky Split Pea and Ham doesn't.

Things get even more confusing when it comes to chicken soups. I've checked some eighteen different varieties of Campbell's chicken soups and found no fewer than ten of them to use margarine, while eight were completely milk free. Do you think I'm going to suggest reading the labels extra carefully? You bet I am.

If you want to play it completely safe, broths and bouillons are your best bets, but there are literally dozens of kinds of soups on the market that are milk free and fine to eat. Making your own "Cream of..." soups isn't that hard either, and I'll give you a recipe later on in Chapter 12.

One final useful bit of information for the soup lover is that while virtually all New England clam chowders are made in a milk base, Manhattan clam chowders use a milk-free tomato base instead.

SURF, TURF, AND CLUCK

No meat, from any animal, contains lactose. The trouble starts once you step away from the fresh meat department and look for the canned meats or the cold cuts or the frozen entrées. Hot dogs often have nonfat dry milk added for filler, although the manufacturers say this in large letters across the front of the package. If you can't find a nice safe brand of kosher hots, then try the "all beef" substitutes instead, as they're more likely to be safe. Precooked hams may be safe, but some "ready to cook" varieties are not. Lots of luncheon meats are extended with milk products.

Canned meats are a good bet, with some exceptions such as chicken stews, which come in a milk-base gravy, and Scalloped Potatoes and Pepperoni, which gives itself away in its name (any food that is "scalloped" contains milk or cream). I was going to advise you to stay away from all spaghetti and meatball variations, because of the added cheese, until I stumbled over Chef Boy Ar Dee's Roller Coasters and Franco-American's PizzO's, miraculously milk free.

And then there're breadings. What's fried chicken without its crisp, crunchy batter? Who could have a fish fry without breaded fish, along with breaded shrimp and breaded clams? (How about some breaded onion rings as a side dish?) Deep-fried breaded mushrooms and cauliflower and broccoli are modern-day appetizers. I've even seen deep-fried pineapple.

Needless to say, wherever there's breading, there's a good chance the bread was made with milk. It ain't necessarily so— for some mysterious reason, it's easier to find frozen breaded clams that are milk free than it is frozen breaded shrimp—but breading ruins a huge number of otherwise useful precooked meat dishes. Tempura batter, however, a Japanese standard now found on frozen fried shrimp and fish, is likely to be milk free. None of this makes up for the disappearance from the market of the last milk-free brand of onion rings I treasured.

As mentioned earlier, the frozen entrée section of the freezer case isn't a good place to look for lactose-free meals. In the old days, TV dinners came with the courses in separate compartments. If you didn't like or couldn't eat one course, you could simply ignore it. Today the meals pretend to come on plates, so even if the meat by itself is okay, the butter sauce on the vegetables will slop over onto it.

I won't even waste my breath on frozen pizzas.

Canned stews (except for chicken stews), hashes, and chilis are usually safe. Tuna fish is healthy and milk free, and sardines are even better, since they are one of the best calcium sources for anyone who can't have milk. Beware the sardines in cream sauces, of course, and be sure to eat the bones.

MISCELLANY

The R. T. French Company makes perfectly safe mustards but adds lactose to its Orange Peel and Lemon Peel. If that doesn't convince you to check the label on every single thing you buy, I don't know what will.

Individual spices should all be okay, but certain blends of spices are not. Watch out for imitation butter flavored extracts as well; not all of them are pure imitations. Monosodium glutamate, the MSG so often found in Chinese cooking, sometimes contains lactose when sold commercially. This doesn't mean that all the MSG in Chinese food is unsafe, but enough people react badly to MSG for one reason or another that I have no hesitation about telling you to avoid it whenever possible.

Another kind of spice blend to beware of is The Salt-Free Alternative, from Estee, which has lactose as an ingredient. Fortunately, there are salt subsitutes that are lactose-free.

Cooked pudding mixes, with the exception of milk chocolate and a few others, are safe, if you can figure out what to add to them in place of the milk; but instant pudding mixes come with the milk already added.

Butter Creme Mint Life Savers use real butter. Butter Rum do not.

Several lactose-free diets warn against corn curls. I've never been able to find any to check. Cheese curls, yes, but you don't need me to tell you to avoid cheese curls. If you run across corn curls, by all means read the ingredients and see what happens.

Very, very few candy bars are completely milk free, unless they are composed entirely of dark or semisweet chocolate. The lack of milk-free sweets in the world is one of the few immediately healthy aspects of a lactose-free diet. Butterless popcorn is a good alternative snack. If you must have sweets, investigate hard candies, licorice, or fruit candies instead.

Sara Lee broke my heart by telling me that all her products contain lactose.

CHAPTER NINE

THE LACTOSE-INTOLERANT CHILD

Babies and milk. The two words associate automatically in our minds, like baseball and hot dogs or rock and roll. Babies are the ultimate milk drinkers everywhere in the world, but we go further in America. Even after baby is weaned, he or she continues to see milk as part of almost every meal, in school lunches, in snacks. Milk and cookies, milk and cereal, milk before bedtime, cheese, ice cream, milk chocolate. Milk drinking may start with babies, but our society makes sure that it continues as the babies grow into children.

Somehow lactose intolerance feels out of place in this idyllic picture. Children should be able to drink milk. But as many parents know, this is not always the case. The ability to drink milk may disappear mysteriously, and reappear later, just as mysteriously. The period when drinking milk leads to diarrhea, cramps, and other complaints may last weeks or months. For a few children, it lasts forever: they are permanently barred from all milk products.

Because of the temporary nature of most of these bouts of milk intolerance, determining the exact cause is not always as important as removing milk from the child's diet. After all, when you're dealing with patients who can't talk, can't pinpoint pains or make

shades of distinction in the way they feel, alleviating the symptoms may be all that is possible without causing worse upsets.
Of course, if milk is reintroduced and still cannot be tolerated,
then tests do need to be run to find out why.

To begin to understand the jumble of problems that can prevent
a child from drinking milk, we need to start even before birth.
Looking at how children develop and the various ills they are
heir to will enable us to sort out a welter of similar-sounding
problems with very different symptoms, as well as some very
different problems with all-too-similar symptoms.

BABIES AND LACTASE

PREMATURE LACTOSE INTOLERANCE AND OTHER CONFUSING TERMS

For the vast majority of babies, worldwide and throughout history,
the first taste of food has been mother's milk, a high-lactose food.
Since not every baby waits a full nine months to be born, you
might expect that babies would be able to manufacture an adequate supply of the lactase enzyme well before birth, in anticipation of that first and crucial meal. For reasons nobody is quite
sure of, however, lactase is one of the *last* digestive enzymes the
fetus begins to manufacture in sufficient quantities to be of much
use.

Lactase activity in the fetus can be detected as early as the
third month of pregnancy. Even so, lactase activity in a six- to
eight-month fetus is only 30 percent what it will be when the
baby is born. Later yet—during the ninth month of pregnancy—
activity is still only 70 percent of the newborn level. This means
that a premature baby weighing three pounds will only absorb
30 to 40 percent of the lactose he or she takes in. A two-pound
premature infant will absorb effectively none. Even some full-
term babies may not produce enough lactase to handle mother's
milk.

Logically, then, all premature babies should suffer the ravaging
symptoms of acute lactose intolerance. To everyone's relief, they
don't. Evidently the first feedings stimulate newborns' bodies to

produce more lactase, allowing them to make efficient use of the milk they're given without becoming ill. Premature infants may fall prey to many problems, but even though it can be shown that the lactose they're drinking is mostly not being absorbed, the symptoms we know as lactose intolerance are usually not among them.

To understand this better, we need to take a closer look at three distinct terms I've been lumping together for the sake of simplicity in this book. *Lactose malabsorption, lactase deficiency*, and *lactose intolerance* are all subtly different conditions, with enough overlap that, for the most part, adults can consider them identical. For babies, however, the differences become more crucial. A newborn baby is almost certainly a lactose malabsorber, may or may not be lactase deficient, but probably doesn't show the symptoms of lactose intolerance.

Lactose malabsorption means simply that lactose is not being well absorbed by the intestines. It can be due to a lack of lactase, or to damaged or incompletely developed intestines. Newborn babies do not have well-developed intestines; even those in full-term babies don't work very efficiently—not nearly as efficiently as they will when the child grows a little older. In addition to this, it takes time for the natural colony of bacteria present in everyone's intestines to grow there, since no bacteria exist in the womb. So while the amount of lactose present in mother's milk may be more than young babies can absorb, the lack of intestinal bacteria ensures that the lactose is not fermented into gas. Instead, the excess lactose is excreted into the stool, providing doctors with an easy test for lactose malabsorption.

Lactase deficiency is a term that applies to all people who do not produce enough lactase to digest milk products in large quantities. Except in a few very rare cases, everyone has sufficient lactose as a child, but most people begin to lose the ability to manufacture lactase as they grow older. Over half the adults in the world are lactase deficient. Most of them don't drink milk or just consume milk products that are very low in lactose, so they aren't aware of any problems. If they were to drink milk, they would wind up with the classic symptoms—diarrhea, gas, cramps—that mark a person as being *lactose intolerant*. Almost everyone who is lactase deficient is potentially lactose intolerant, so most people use the terms interchangeably. A lucky few, however, test out as being mildly lactase deficient but still get no symptoms even when given a lactose load.

In practical terms, parents have little need to worry about the ailment in newborns called premature lactose intolerance. Some premature infants do suffer from lactose malabsorption, but the symptoms of lactose intolerance will be short-lived, if they occur at all. After the very first few months of your baby's life, it's the lactose intolerance you have to worry about, since without the symptoms, there is no cause for alarm, even if tests show lactase deficiency or lactose malabsorption.

LACTOSE INTOLERANCE IN OLDER CHILDREN

Older here means any child past the newborn stage, say, from about nine months on up. Gas, cramps, and short-term diarrhea are hardly unusual symptoms in children, even in otherwise healthy children. Only if these symptoms stay on and on and never go away are they a matter of concern for a doctor (although you as parents may have long since been frantic with worry). Such chronic diarrhea—the short-term variety is called acute diarrhea—may involve attacks of watery diarrhea four to six times a day. Gas and stomach pain are normal when this happens, and so is an irritated bottom—lactose intolerance produces an acidic stool.

These few symptoms should be enough to make your doctor think of lactose intolerance. Other diagnoses are still possible at this point, some of them even milk related. If the baby is a newborn, the doctor may consider galactosemia or glucose-galactose malabsorption. Children at any age may show these symptoms because of a milk protein allergy, although if this is the problem, they usually have several other symptoms as well. (See Chapter 4 for information on these ailments.)

To make a diagnosis, your doctor may order a whole battery of tests (the ones mentioned in Chapter 3). Or no tests may be run at all.

If your doctor doesn't do any testing, that doesn't necessarily mean that it's time to get a new doctor. There are good reasons for not doing tests. For one thing, the tests are likely to make a small ailing child even more uncomfortable than before. A large dose of lactose, followed by six blood samples, the form of one common test, can be a painful experience even for an adult suffering from lactose intolerance.

Not all the tests cause such problems, however. One test especially useful for very small children is checking the stool for acidity and lactose, high quantities of which point to lactose intolerance. This test is more an indirect way of inferring lactose intolerance than a proof, however. If the facilities are available, then a hydrogen breath test should be run. As described in Chapter 3, this test (originally developed for babies) doesn't require any tubes or needles and is extremely accurate in predicting lactose intolerance.

Either way, tests or no tests, the question of whether lactose intolerance is the cause of your child's symptoms is usually settled in the most straightforward manner: putting the child on a lactose-free diet. Depending upon the age of the child, such a diet may mean one of the soy formulas available on the market, or just a junior version of the lactose-free diet an adult would eat. For in-betweeners, all the major baby food companies make a variety of foods that are lactose-free.

In adults, lactose intolerance that comes from the normal loss of lactase in aging is called primary lactose intolerance. Having a disease knock out the ability of the intestines to manufacture lactose is called secondary lactose intolerance. Children get both types as well, though they are called by other names. Developmental lactose intolerance results, like primary, from the loss of lactase through natural processes. Acquired lactose intolerance, like secondary, hits after the intestines have been affected by a disease powerful enough to stop lactase production.

In children, however, these two causes tend to be jumbled together, making it very difficult to tell one from the other. It's natural to gradually lose the ability to produce lactase. If more than half the adults alive in the world today have lactose intolerance (a conservative figure), then well over a billion adults have seen their lactase production drop. For some of them, it must certainly have happened as children.

Among cultures where all the adults are lactose intolerant, for example in Thailand or among the Pima Indians, the children stop being able to digest milk by the age of four. Nobody is really sure what the comparable age is for Americans. One study found that three-quarters of American black eight- and nine-year-olds tested were lactose intolerant and that 20 percent of white schoolchildren of the same age were.

Even these studies can only say what has already happened to a large group. If your particular four- or eight-year-old suddenly starts becoming intolerant to milk, who's to say whether this indicates the beginning of a steady drop in lactase or just the aftereffect of a bad intestinal flu? Doctors certainly can't. Another study examined children diagnosed as lactose intolerant three to five months after the original diagnosis. A full 40 percent of the group were having no trouble at all with lactose when the follow-up study was completed.

Because of this uncertainty, there's a very good chance that the lactose-free diet your child goes on may not have to be permanent. Even children destined to be lactose-intolerant adults may have just had their lactase production dropped to zero by a particularly nasty flu. After the disease runs its course, the lactase may come back.

For this reason, pediatricians say that you should cautiously reintroduce milk into your child's diet after dropping it for several months. The odds are good that he or she will have no trouble digesting it at all. (Ironically, the trouble may be that your child, having gotten used to the taste of soy or other substitutes, no longer likes the taste of real milk. You should be able to get around this fairly easily.)

Unlike some of the more common childhood diseases, like measles, getting acquired lactose intolerance doesn't give you any immunity from suffering from it again and again. If your child gets a series of three or four bad intestinal flus, then his or her lactase production may be knocked out three or four times. Other intestinal complaints or operations may do the same thing. Going on and off milk may be nerve-wracking for you, your child, and your whole family, but it's far better than the intolerance symptoms would be.

Other Signs of Lactose Intolerance

Adults with different degrees of lactose intolerance can show a spectrum of symptoms, so why should children be different? Sometimes, especially when the child has developmental lactose intolerance, the symptoms will be gas and pain along with constipation, but no diarrhea. The symptoms will generally appear two to four hours after having lactose, say around noontime because of breakfast milk, or just after bedtime if milk is drunk with dinner. In this case as well, the best way to find out if lactose intolerance is the problem is to cut out all milk and milk products for a while. If the symptoms go away, then lactose intolerance was the culprit. If not, see your doctor.

A far more serious problem is known as recurrent abdominal pain (RAP). Somewhere between 9 and 15 percent of children suffer from RAP, pain that is serious enough to disrupt a child's activities and that recurs a number of times over a period of months. Some cases may last even longer, with a large number of RAP victims missing more than one day of school out of every ten.

Traditionally doctors either have tried to identify a standard physical cause for the pain, ordering test after test to exclude all the known intestinal complaints, or have tried to associate the problem with behavioral or personality disorders. Recently, since the traditional methods accomplished little more than running up huge medical bills (one group of 119 RAP patients had undergone 225 different major tests), doctors have begun to investigate whether unsuspected lactose intolerance might be a root cause.

The results have been mixed. One study found that 40 percent of the RAP victims examined were not absorbing lactose properly, and 70 percent of these had more pain attacks on a diet containing lactose than on a lactose-free diet. Other studies have had even better success in removing pain with a low-lactose diet. Still, the majority of the children studied did not have lactose intolerance and got no better on a lactose-free diet. Later studies have also dashed hopes by stating that lactose malabsorption and RAP are two different things, and that a low-lactose diet may alleviate symptoms due to lactose intolerance but does not present a cure for RAP. While any child with RAP should experiment with a lactose-free diet, the treatment is obviously no cure-all.

CONGENITAL LACTOSE INTOLERANCE

Every once in a blue moon, a baby is born without any lactase whatsoever. It's such an extremely rare condition that a pediatrician at a busy hospital may see only a single case in a professional lifetime.

Congenital lactose intolerance is as serious as it is unusual. Symptoms include diarrhea, vomiting, distension, and irritability after the first few feedings. If the cause is not guessed and the infant continues to drink milk, the result can be devastating. Water loss through diarrhea can lead to dehydration, the chronic diarrhea itself may cause malabsorption of other nutrients, and severe malnutrition is a possibility. All this can be fatal if not stopped in time.

Today, with the symptoms of lactose intolerance so widely recognized, it's not likely that any doctor would let a baby suffer for so long. It's known that violent symptoms of this type are associated with milk reactions, so milk feedings would be stopped immediately, even before anybody attempted to determine which milk reaction was the exact cause. (Other problems, like glucose-galactose malabsorption, could have exactly the same set of symptoms.)

True congenital lactose intolerance is permanent and irreversible. All that can be done is to put the infant onto a soy formula until he or she is old enough to start on a lactose-free diet of solid foods.

LACTOSE INTOLERANCE AND THE MILK DRINKER

Since drinking milk makes many children sick, you might think that children or their parents would make the association and give up drinking milk by themselves. Maybe some do, but many don't. In the study of RAP victims I talked about above, the doctors found there was no difference in milk drinking, frequency of pain, or presence or absence of diarrhea between the group of lactose malabsorbers and the group of absorbers.

If you go on to look at other studies, you can find evidence
to prove a case either way. One of the classic studies that first
demonstrated the extent of milk intolerance among minority children in this country showed that black schoolchildren failed to
finish their school lunch milk far more often than white schoolchildren. Blacks have a much higher incidence of lactose intolerance than whites and develop it an earlier age, so that result
makes sense. But when you look at black absorbers versus black
malabsorbers, milk drinking is exactly the same. And so it goes,
with one set of researchers saying one thing and another set
something else.

Age has a lot to do with it, as well. Younger children, those
three or four years of age, are often very proud of learning that
they are somehow special by not being able to drink milk. They'll
often stop anyone trying to offer them a cookie or candy by
saying very forthrightly, No, I can't have it. Once children get
into school, being different is something they would rather hide.
Most lactose-intolerant children go through phases in which they'll
try milk, even if they know they'll pay for it later with a stomach-
ache or diarrhea. Ice cream is the hardest thing for them to give
up.

How bad their symptoms are will play a major role in whether
they're going to try milk or not. One study of children found that
80 percent of those with severe lactose intolerance said they were
going to stay away from milk in the future, but a full 97 percent
of those with mild intolerance said they would have milk again.

Keeping your lactose-intolerant child on a lactose-free diet at
home is always a good idea. Depending upon how severe the
symptoms are, an occasional lapse from a strictly milk-free diet
so that he or she can take part in the same activities as everyone
else might not be a bad idea. Be sure to have an ample supply
of one of the lactase tablets or capsules on hand to keep the
symptoms down afterward, though.

One thing you can do is spread the word through your friends
and family. There's no reason a visit to grandma's house or an
overnight stay at a friend's has to be an exercise in avoiding
temptation. Lots of snacks and goodies either come lactose-free
in the first place or can easily be made in lactose-free form at

home, using the milk-free substitutes that I talk about in Chapter 6. Giving children some of these to eat during the visit rather than having them eat whatever happens to be set in front of them by their host or hostess will save a lot of trouble and pain afterward. Providing milk-free recipes to the parents of your child's friends will give them an easy way out if they're not sure what to serve.

If your child is one of those who develops a permanent lactose intolerance at an early age, you'll have to teach him or her how to say no. A polite "I'm sorry, but I can't eat that" will deflect a lot of potentially troublesome food. Neither you nor they will be able to guard against all food all the time, but making them aware of the problem and of the consequences will give them the strength and the ammunition to fend off a lot of well-intentioned but ignorant adults.

LACTOSE-FREE INFANT FORMULAS

NUTRITION

The use of soybean "milk" as a substitute for cow's milk in infant feeding dates all the way back to 1909. Today's infants have a much better selection of formulas—healthier, tastier, and devised for just about any intestinal problems they may have.

Any milk substitutes for infants should fulfill all the following criteria:

1. contain protein, fat, and carbohydrate in amounts roughly similar to those in human milk, along with an adequate supply of vitamins and minerals
2. be as low-allergenic as possible
3. be easy to prepare
4. taste and smell good enough that infants will drink enough to stay healthy
5. be readily available at a reasonable price

To meet these criteria, manufacturers take very much the same paths, varying only in the details. The major brands in the field (and their makers) are ProSobee (Mead Johnson), Nursoy (Wyeth),

Isomil (Ross), Soyalac (Loma Linda), and Mull-Soy Liquid (Borden). As several of the names imply, all are variations on soybean "milks." Your doctor may recommend one over the other because of personal preferences or your own child's special case, but if not, any of these should be acceptable milk substitutes.

The small differences among them may be worth considering, however, depending upon whatever other ailments your child might have. Some lactose-intolerant children also have milk protein allergy. Children with one allergy seem to be more prone to acquiring additional allergies, so formulas with the lowest likelihood of causing an allergic reaction may be preferred. Isomil, ProSobee, and Nursoy all use soy protein isolate rather than soy flour as their protein source. Soy-protein isolate has been heat treated to be less allergenic.

Although all five formulas are free of lactose, they all include other sugars for their carbohydrate value. Some boast of having no corn syrup, others of containing no sucrose (table sugar). A few children have corn allergies, and I know many parents are striving to keep their children away from table sugar, so check with your doctor to see if any of this makes a difference in your child's case.

Most children thrive on a diet of these formulas even when they drink nothing else (although when your child is six months of age, you should start adding other foods to the diet). Studies have shown that infants grow just as much on soy-based formulas as they do on milk-based formulas, and that they don't develop a large number of feeding problems.

In addition, the nutrient value of these formulas has been improved and refined over the years to be closely comparable to mother's milk and cow's milk. All the major formulas, in fact, contain even more calcium than does mother's milk, so you don't have to worry about your child missing that extremely important mineral so vital to developing healthy bones and teeth in a growing child.

Still, the one flaw in all these formulas is their soy base. As many as one-fourth of milk-sensitive babies become allergic to soy protein after long exposure to it.

Mead Johnson makes two infant formulas without soy for infants with this problem: Nutramigen and Pregestimil. Both use enzymically hydrolyzed casein, or cow's protein, as their protein source. *Enzymically hydrolyzed* means "digested," so the casein is virtually allergic free and essentially lactose free. In their other nutrients, these two formulas are quite close to the soy-based lactose-free formulas.

Few other choices exist for infants who cannot tolerate any of these formulas. Gerber used to make Lambase and MBF (Meat-Based Formula), which were often recommended in older books, but both have been withdrawn from the market. One other possible option, though not normally thought of as an infant formula, is Vivonex (Eaton), a so-called elemental formula. This formula has no plant or animal proteins; all the protein it contains is synthetic. Vivonex is tolerated well by milk-sensitive patients who can't use any of the other milk substitutes.

FEEDING

These formulas come in a variety of different forms, of varying convenience. The most common types are

- Powder: the most concentrated and cheapest.
- Ready-to-use: most expensive (because you are paying for the company's shipping and storing water) but also most convenient because it can be used straight out of the can.
- Concentrated liquid: midway between the other two in price and convenience; typically you add 1 part water to 1 part formula.

Formula should be prepared strictly according to its manufacturer's instructions, but once prepared, feeding your child with it is no different than any other bottle-feeding.

After the Bottle

After your child outgrows bottle-feedings, the formulas can also be used in place of milk in preparing lactose-free meals. Some experience is necessary to cook with them; a few of the formulas have a tendency to separate in heating. Still, they make a useful bridge between the bottle years and the time when your child is ready to use an adult milk substitute.

Using these formulas for cooking has another advantage in that they are far healthier and have many more nutrients than the Coffee Rich–type milk substitutes. Using them along with a good balanced diet should provide all the vitamins and minerals your child will normally need. (The Recommended Daily Allowances for vitamins and minerals can be found in the next chapter.)

If you choose not to use these formulas in cooking, and your child is on a completely milk-free diet, you still have little need to worry. A good balanced diet, high in the foods that supply the vitamins and minerals normally found in milk, as outlined in Chapter 10, will prevent serious problems. Ask your doctor if a calcium supplement or children's vitamins are recommended in your child's case.

CHAPTER TEN

HEALTH, WELL-BEING, AND THE CAREFUL CONSUMER

Few of us have a perfect diet, and with half the most tempting foods in the world stuffed with lactose, most of us are going to wind up falling off the lactose wagon. For most of us, that means a day or two of feeling lousy, at the very least.

This chapter will look at both sides of health: living healthily and recovering health when you lose it. We'll start with the basics of nutrition and the nutrients you lose by not drinking milk. Following that is a section on soothing the most common ailments associated with lactose intolerance: gas, diarrhea, and hemorrhoids. In closing, I'll also talk about the health risks of finding lactose in the worst possible place—in medication.

HEALTH: WITH AND WITHOUT MILK

If you can drink milk, you should. You need it. I have to say this because milk won its case in court.

Back in the 1970s, the California Milk Producers Advisory

Board sponsored a famous set of commercials using celebrities such as Mark Spitz and Dear Abby to push the slogan, Every Body Needs Milk. The Federal Trade Commission took a look around at all of us with lactose intolerance and milk allergies and said, essentially, "That's not true. Change your slogan." They all wound up in court.

After 12,919 transcript pages, fourteen volumes of exhibits, and thirty-five witnesses, Administrative Law Judge Daniel H. Hanscom presented the world with a 120-page opinion that is one of the best summaries we have of the role of milk in American nutrition and the problems of the lactose intolerant.

All in all, the hearings in this case confirmed the fact that milk is critically important in our society. The judge wrote, "Milk is one of the most nutritious foods in this nation's diet, and from the standpoint of the population as a whole, or even significant population groups, is literally 'essential, necessary and needed.' The withdrawal of milk from any major population group would amount to nutritional disaster."

At the same time, the expert witnesses, who included many of the doctors whose names appear over and over on articles on lactose intolerance in the medical journals, provided evidence that, for the first time in such a public forum, brought home the magnitude of the problem of lactose intolerance. Judge Hanscom acknowledged that we do, indeed, have special problems, writing, "It was unfair and misleading for respondents to represent to lactase deficient persons, who constitute a substantial segment of the population, that the consumption of large or unlimited quantities of milk at a time is beneficial."

In the end, Judge Hanscom threw out the FTC complaint on the grounds that "Ingestion of large or unlimited amounts of milk at one time by such persons [the lactose intolerant] may cause problems which are troublesome or discomforting, although not health threatening." In other words, if it doesn't kill you, I can't help you.

Milk continues to be advertised, though the slogan was eventually changed to Milk Has Something For Every Body, which is impossible to argue with. Does giving up milk mean a "nutritional disaster," as the judge wrote? Of course not. I'm probably healthier now than I was while I was still drinking milk, because overall my diet is better. We need to take a close look at milk so that you can decide whether to give it up entirely or whether you're willing to drink enough to force you to decide just how "troublesome or discomforting" your problems have to get before the disadvantages of milk outweigh its many pluses.

Before I get to the specific nutrients milk provides, I want you to be aware of the nutrient labeling on many packaged foods, an essential to understanding a balanced diet in the absence of milk.

NUTRITION LABELING

Unlike ingredients lists, which are required on all packaged foods, nutrition information is required only on enriched or fortified foods or those that make a nutritional claim, such as "high protein" or "low calorie." For all other foods, nutrition labels are voluntary.

Nutrition labels come in several variations, but the most usual one, and the one with the best information, contains the following:

- the serving size and number of servings per container
- the number of calories per serving
- the number of grams of protein, carbohydrate, and fat per serving (there are 28 grams to an ounce and 454 grams to one pound)
- the percentage of the U.S. Adult Recommended Daily Allowance (RDA) per serving for eight important nutrients—protein, vitamin A, vitamin C, thiamin, riboflavin, niacin, calcium, and iron—which happen to include many of the ones milk is especially high in

The U.S. RDA causes a great deal of unnecessary confusion. Many people worry if they're not getting a full 100 percent of the RDA of every nutrient every day. It can't hurt you to reach the 100 percent value, but the RDA is set higher than most people ever need. In fact, the RDA for adults is based on the group (other than pregnant and nursing women) with the highest need for each nutrient. The RDA for adults for thiamin, a vitamin, is 1.5 milligrams. Only teenage males need a full 1.5. Women over the age of fifty only need 70 percent of this amount. On the other

Food and Nutrition Board, National Academy of Sciences–National Research Council Recommended Daily Dietary Allowances, Revised 1980

Designed for the maintenance of good nutrition of practically all healthy people in the U.S.A.

	AGE (years)	WEIGHT (kg)	WEIGHT (lb)	HEIGHT (cm)	HEIGHT (in)	PROTEIN (g)	VITAMIN A (μg RE)[b]	VITAMIN D (μg)[c]	VITAMIN E (mg α-TE)[d]	VITAMIN C (mg)	THIAMIN (mg)
							FAT-SOLUBLE VITAMINS				
Infants	0.0–0.5	6	13	60	24	kg. × 2.2	420	10	3	35	0.3
	0.5–1.0	9	20	71	28	kg. × 2.0	400	10	4	35	0.5
Children	1–3	13	29	90	35	23	400	10	5	45	0.7
	4–6	20	44	112	44	30	500	10	6	45	0.9
	7–10	28	62	132	52	34	700	10	7	45	1.2
Males	11–14	45	99	157	62	45	1000	10	8	50	1.4
	15–18	66	145	176	69	56	1000	10	10	60	1.4
	19–22	70	154	177	70	56	1000	7.5	10	60	1.5
	23–50	70	154	178	70	56	1000	5	10	60	1.4
	51 +	70	154	178	70	56	1000	5	10	60	1.2
Females	11–14	46	101	157	62	46	800	10	8	50	1.1
	15–18	55	120	163	64	46	800	10	8	60	1.1
	19–22	55	120	163	64	44	800	7.5	8	60	1.1
	23–50	55	120	163	64	44	800	5	8	60	1.0
	51 +	55	120	163	64	44	800	5	8	60	1.0
Pregnant						+30	+200	+5	+2	+20	+0.4
Lactating						+20	+400	+5	+3	+40	+0.4

SOURCE: National Research Council.

[a] The allowances are intended to provide for individual variations among most normal persons as they live in the United States under usual environmental stresses. Diets should be based on a variety of common foods in order to provide other nutrients for which human requirements have been less well defined.

[b] Retinol equivalents. 1 retinol equivalent = 1 μg retinol or 6 μg β carotene.

[c] As cholecalciferol. 10 μg cholecalciferol = 400 IU of vitamin D.

[d] α-tocopherol equivalents. 1 mg d-α tocopherol = 1 α-TE.

[e] 1 NE (niacin equivalent) is equal to 1 mg of niacin or 60 mg of dietary tryptophan.

[f] The folacin allowances refer to dietary sources as determined by *Lactobacillus casei* assay after treatment with enzymes (conjugases) to make polyglutamyl

					MINERALS					
RIBO-FLAVIN (mg)	NIACIN (mg NE)^r	VITA-MIN B-6 (mg)	FOLA-CIN^f (μg)	VITAMIN B-12 (μg)	CAL-CIUM (mg)	PHOS-PHORUS (mg)	MAG-NESIUM (mg)	IRON (mg)	ZINC (mg)	IODINE (μg)
0.4	6	0.3	30	0.5	360	240	50	10	3	40
0.6	8	0.6	45	1.5	540	360	70	15	5	50
0.8	9	0.9	100	2.0	800	800	150	15	10	70
1.0	11	1.3	200	2.5	800	800	200	10	10	90
1.4	16	1.6	300	3.0	800	800	250	10	10	120
1.6	18	1.8	400	3.0	1200	1200	350	18	15	150
1.7	18	2.0	400	3.0	1200	1200	400	18	15	150
1.7	19	2.2	400	3.0	800	800	350	10	15	150
1.6	18	2.2	400	3.0	800	800	350	10	15	150
1.4	16	2.2	400	3.0	800	800	350	10	15	150
1.3	15	1.8	400	3.0	1200	1200	300	18	15	150
1.3	14	2.0	400	3.0	1200	1200	300	18	15	150
1.3	14	2.0	400	3.0	800	800	300	18	15	150
1.2	13	2.0	400	3.0	800	800	300	18	15	150
1.2	13	2.0	400	3.0	800	800	300	10	15	150
+0.3	+2	+0.6	+400	+1.0	+400	+400	+150	h	+5	+25
+0.3	+5	+0.5	+100	+1.0	+400	+400	+150	h	+10	+50

forms of the vitamin available to the test organism.

^{g} The recommended dietary alowance for vitamin B12 in infants is based on averge concentrtion of the vitmain in human milk. The allowances after weaning are based on energy intake (as recommended by the American Academy of Pediatrics) and consideration of other factors, such as intestinal absorption.

^{h} The increased requirement during pregnancy cannot be met by the iron content of habitual American diets or by the existing iron stores of man women; therefore the use of 30–60 mg of supplemental iron is recommended. Iron needs during lactation are not substantially different from those of nonpregnant women, but continued supplementation ofthe mother for 2–3 months after parturition is advisable in order to replenish storesdepleted by pregnancy.

hand, pregnant and nursing women almost always need far more than 100 percent of the RDA for any nutrient. Infants, children, adult males, and adult females each have their own very different sets of RDAs.

One other bit of confusion is that *adult* is defined as anyone over the age of eleven, but teenagers and grown-ups can have different RDAs. Later on in this chapter, when I talk about adult RDAs, I'll be referring to adults over the age of twenty-three, not teenagers, unless specifically mentioned.

When planning meals and looking for foods that will supply the nutrients otherwise obtained from milk, it's not always necessary to hit 100 percent of the RDA. The preceding chart, prepared by the National Academy of Sciences–National Research Council's Food and Nutrition Board, shows you how much you need to shoot for.

Nutrient Density

Milk is unique in our diet because it contains about 100 nutrients, or virtually every nutrient known. Even better, it contains many of them in important quantities, important because nutrients interact with one another and so require one another's presence to work properly in our bodies.

Even for adults, milk is valuable because it has a high nutrient density. High nutrient density foods are low in calories, low in fats and sugars, and high in vitamins, minerals, and protein—all the things nutritionists say you should be eating. Milk is a perfect high density food because it contains so much that is good and so little of the fats and sugars that are considered to be bad.

You can easily determine for yourself the nutrient density of packaged foods using their nutrition labels (assuming they're the type that lists protein, vitamin A, vitamin C, thiamin, riboflavin, niacin, calcium, and iron):

1. Add the total percentage of the U.S. RDA per serving for the eight nutrients listed on a nutrition label.
2. Divide this total by the number of calories in that serving.
3. Multiply the result by 100.

For example:

RDA PERCENTAGE PER SERVING:	DEVILS FOOD CAKE MIX	FROZEN SPINACH
Protein	2	4
Vitamin A	less than 2%	150
Vitamin C	less than 2%	35
Thiamin	4	6
Riboflavin	2	8
Niacin	2	less than 2%
Calcium	2	10
Iron	8	10
Total	20	223
Calories per-serving	180	20
Nutrient adensity:	$20/180 \times 100 = 11$	$223/20 \times 100 = 1,115$

No wonder Popeye always bests Bluto. Spinach beats the cake mix in seven of the eight nutrients, showing a good balance across the field, though it's the phenomenal vitamin A score that boosts spinach so high. The fact that a cake mix is incomplete doesn't affect its nutrient density. Adding water, one-third cup of vegetable oil, and three eggs to make the finished cake does not change the nutrient density at all, since the extra nutrient value is balanced by a proportionate number of calories.

A sampling of nutrient density scores from the packages on my kitchen shelves: brown rice—13; chicken noodle soup—29; frozen sweet corn—43; wheat cereal—123; frozen broccoli—624. Whole milk's score varies somewhat depending upon the percentage of fat included but winds up in the high 70s. This means adding milk to the wheat cereal actually lowers the final score, to 100.

Nutrient density scores are, at best, guidelines and warnings. There's nothing wrong with brown rice, despite its low score—although a diet consisting solely of brown rice would be a disaster. For that matter, you can't live on any one food, no matter how high the nutrient density score; imagine eating nothing but spinach morning, noon, and night. If you could eat that much spinach, the high vitamin A score wouldn't make up for the low levels of protein or niacin, thiamin, and riboflavin. No single food is perfect.

Milk's medium-level score shouldn't disguise the fact that it offers a good balance of nutrients (including some not listed on the label) and very high quality protein. Very low scores, on the other hand, are warnings. You won't find nutrition labeling on soft drinks because their manufacturers don't want to admit that the nutrient density of a soft drink is essentially zero. The real purpose of the scores to us is to provide one more valuable guideline for creating a diet containing sufficient quantities of the nutrients lost by not having milk.

Because milk contains a good balance of nutrients and is easily available everywhere (and because it's so much easier to drink large quantities of milk than to eat any amount of spinach), milk products are a mainstay of most adults' diets, thereby supplying most Americans with a great many of the nutrients they need. A study conducted by the Department of Agriculture in 1977 found that although dairy foods (excluding butter) contributed only 11 percent of the calories in American diets, they provided 22 percent of the protein and large quantities of important minerals, including 35 percent of the phosphorus, 22 percent of the magnesium, and a whopping 75 percent of the calcium intake. Major amounts of vitamins, including 39 percent of the riboflavin, 20 percent of the vitamin B_{12}, and 13 percent of the vitamin A also come from the dairy food group.

Except for calcium, it's relatively easy to make up for the loss of these percentages by increasing your intake of other foods that are high in these vitamins and minerals. Unfortunately, since every person's diet is different, I can't say just how much more of those foods to eat. By paying close attention and making sure that your diet is rich in these foods, and taking vitamin and mineral supplements if you want to be positive you're getting an adequate supply, you should have no worries about not eating milk products. Calcium is a special case, and I'll discuss calcium supplements later in this chapter.

In the next section, I'll discuss exactly what these nutrients do and what alternative sources for them exist. Protein's importance to the body was outlined in Chapter 2. Since most meats, seafood, grains, and legumes (peas and beans) are good, if sometimes incomplete, sources of protein, the average American's diet is awash in protein, more than is necessary for health. While the protein in milk is very high quality, only a badly unbalanced milk-free diet could cause a protein deficiency.

The specific vitamins and minerals that are mentioned here are covered in the next sections.

Calcium

The vast majority of calcium in the average American's diet comes from milk products, making it the hardest nutrient to acquire without milk.

The role of calcium in our lives is obvious: 99 percent of the calcium in the body is in our bones and teeth. The other 1 percent has important roles in blood clotting, nerve stimulation, muscle tone, enzyme activation, and vitamin absorption. Lack of calcium can result in bone malformation, causing both the children's disease known as rickets and osteomalacia, a bone disorder in adults. A rapidly increasing health problem among older women is osteoporosis, which is enough of a concern that I'll devote a special section to it right after this one.

Calcium absorption by the body is very inefficient. Only about 20 to 30 percent of the calcium we eat actually gets used. If you eat foods containing 800 milligrams of calcium in a day, your body will only absorb about 200 milligrams. Ironically, the lactose in milk increases calcium absorption by 15 to 20 percent, so not only do lactose-intolerant people get less calcium by not drinking milk, they also capture and use less efficiently what calcium they do get in their diet.

Calcium absorption also depends upon the presence of vitamin D and phosphorus. Vitamin D enhances absorption of calcium from the digestive tract. Phosphorus forms with calcium the mineral compounds actually deposited in bones.

Most adults and children require 800 milligrams of calcium in their diet every day. Teenagers should get even more—around 1200 milligrams, the same as pregnant or lactating women.

No other food is as good a source of calcium as milk, which provides 228 milligrams of calcium per 8-ounce glass; the other foods that are relatively high in calcium are ones that few people eat large amounts of: green leafy vegetables, peas, dried beans, tofu or tempeh, and canned fish (as long as you eat the bones) are the best alternative sources. Unfortunately, many of the green leafy vegetables, including spinach, rhubarb, chard, beet tops, and parsley, contain a substance called oxalic acid, which combines with calcium and interferes with its absorption. Oxylates can even form kidney stones or gallstones. Other foods with oxalic acid are cocoa, tea, almonds, and cashews. High-protein diets, high-fiber diets, and high-fat diets may also interfere with calcium absorption.

In fact, it's so hard to get enough usable calcium without milk that calcium supplements are necessary for virtually everyone on a milk-free or low-milk diet. Most supplements contain calcium in the form of calcium carbonate, since that provides the highest usable amount of calcium per pill. Calcium lactate, calcium phosphate, and calcium gluconate are also sometimes used, especially since large amounts of calcium carbonate can cause constipation or gas. Calcium chloride is not recommended, since it can irritate the stomach lining. Pure calcium is never used, since it will not be absorbed well by the body.

Lately there has been a great deal of controversy over which is the best form of calcium supplement to take. Most sources agree that dolomite and bone meal are to be avoided, as samples have been found to be contaminated with lead and other toxic metals. Oyster-shell calcium pills are relatively inexpensive and are lead free, but one study did find trace amounts of heavy metals.

Tums, the over-the-counter antacid, has been recommended as an inexpensive calcium supplement because Tums are mostly calcium carbonate. (Other antacids contain aluminum, which can remove calcium from the body.) Tums will certainly work—calcium carbonate is calcium carbonate—but I have my doubts whether Tums is a good source of calcium, although, if bought in large enough quantities, it is inexpensive. A roll of 12 Tums, each providing 200 milligrams of calcium, costs 45 cents. A jar of 150, bought on sale in a local store, costs $2.34. That means a day's supply of calcium, 800 milligrams, costs you between 6 and 15 cents. National brand calcium supplements such as Os-Cal (from Marion), Posture (Ayerst Labs), BioCal (Miles Labs), and Caltrate (Lederle Labs) cost about 15 to 20 cents for a daily dose when you buy them at regular prices, but you can often find the supplements discounted in drugstores and supermarkets, saving you money. Better yet, they lack the flavorings and additives Tums has and you don't need.

If you want to take a calcium supplement, be sure to take one that comes with vitamim D in the pill to help with the absorption of the calcium (something Tums lacks). These pills are somewhat more expensive than the straight calcium supplements, but worth the extra cost.

I don't like to recommend particular brands when a number of choices of equal quality exist, but I'll make an exception in this case. Caltrate 600 + Vitamin D says right on its label, "No Lactose." It's good consumerism to support those companies that support the lactose intolerant.

Osteoporosis

The hardness of our bones is largely a matter of density: the minerals that make up the bones are tightly packed into a small space. Like the other systems in our bodies, bones are in a state of equilibrium. The mineral content in bones is constantly being lost and replaced, to maintain a proper balance both in the bones and in the other systems where the minerals are needed. As we grow older, bone formation stops making up for bone loss. To keep the calcium levels high in the crucial nerve centers, calcium is drawn out of the spongy inner layers of bone. A woman reaching her ninetieth birthday will have lost 43 percent of this inner layer. Bones lose their density, become brittle. This is quite normal. When the process goes too far, it turns into a disease.

Osteo relates to bones; *porosis* refers to being porous. But osteoporosis is more than the normal state of porous bones. Having the disease means that so much of the bones has been lost that the skeleton can no longer support the body properly. Fractures become common; about 1.3 million fractures are attributed to osteoporosis each year. In fact, complications resulting from bone fracture are the third leading cause of death in people over sixty-five.

Osteoporosis is far more prevalant in women than men and far more common in whites than in blacks, though even black males can develop it. One in three women and one in five men between the ages of forty-five and seventy-five have osteoporosis, and their numbers are increasing every year, both because people, and especially women, are living longer and because our lifestyles predispose us to osteoporosis.

Women are at especial risk for a number of reasons: They start with less bone than do men, they have rapid bone loss beginning at menopause, and their diets are lower in calcium, on the average, than men's. Factors other than gender also come into play. Alcoholism, smoking, high caffeine intake and high-protein diets, lack of exercise, and general poor nutrition all increase your risk of having osteoporosis.

Even with a good diet and proper exercise, your body's efficiency in absorbing calcium, never very high to begin with, decreases with age, starting at age forty-five in women and age sixty in men. The lactose intolerant are doubly hurt, as I previously mentioned, since we get neither the calcium from milk products nor the boost that lactose gives to calcium absorption. This makes the lactose intolerant a special high-risk group when it comes to getting osteoporosis.

Serious osteoporosis is, of course, a matter for a doctor's care. Doctors often recommend an increase in calcium to 1000 or even 1500 milligrams a day, along with additional vitamin D and magnesium. Large doses of any of these can cause side effects, so the levels you take have to be monitored carefully.

One other course of treatment is estrogen therapy. Estrogen is a hormone lost after women go through menopause, and replacing the estrogen seems to reduce bone loss. However, estrogen therapy is still unproved and very controversial, associated with even worse side effects than are large doses of calcium, and strictly for a doctor to prescribe.

Osteoporosis is much like lactose intolerance in that it affects millions of Americans, many of whom have never even heard of the disorder, and in that the magnitude and seriousness of the problem is just beginning to be recognized. It's a key reason an adequate daily supply of calcium is crucial to everyone with lactose intolerance. Female readers should be doubly sure to get more information on osteoporosis, while older females would do well to check in with a doctor just to play it safe.

PHOSPHORUS

Every cell, living or once living, has some phosphorus, so it is supplied by all plant and animal foods. Meat, poultry, fish, eggs, and whole-grain cereals are especially high in the mineral. Phosphorus combines with calcium to build bones and ideally should be taken one-for-one with calcium (except for infants, who need twice as much phosphorus as calcium). On the other hand, too much phosphorus can demineralize bones, causing a need for even more calcium, which is no longer being used efficiently.

The adult and child RDA for phosphorus is exactly the same as it is for calcium. The problem is that the standard American diet has too much phosphorus and too little calcium in it. Although phosphorus is easily available (from soft drinks especially), and efficiently absorbed (50 to 70 percent), its absorption and usefulness depend on the presence of vitamin D and calcium. Rather than trying to cut down on phosphorus—a difficult task—it's better to make sure that you're getting an adequate supply of calcium. If the calcium-phosphorus balance is upset, arthritis, rickets, or tooth decay may result.

MAGNESIUM

Magnesium is found in all parts of the body, but 70 percent of the body's supply is in the bones, along with the body's calcium and phosphorus. Calcium and magnesium need to be balanced, with magnesium intake rising as calcium intake increases. Magnesium is also necessary for crucial enzymes, proteins, and hormones to function.

Plant foods are the best sources of magnesium. Whole grains are rich in the mineral, but milling removes it. Other good sources are nuts, dried beans, green plants and vegetables, coffee, and cocoa.

The RDA for magnesium is 350 milligrams for adult males, 400 for adult females, 450 for pregnant or nursing women. The average diet just barely supplies enough for normal adults, so the loss of milk is bound to cause a deficiency. Besides, the cooking of food will remove magnesium, and oxalic acid works to bind magnesium in the same way it binds calcium.

Magnesium deficiency can occur in patients with many diseases, including diabetes, alcoholism, and cirrhosis of the liver. Some studies have related it to coronary heart disease. In addition, the need for magnesium increases when blood cholesterol levels are high and when consumption of protein is high.

RIBOFLAVIN

Riboflavin is the chemical name for vitamin B_2. It's found in most foods, but milk products are the only ones that are both high in riboflavin and eaten in large quantities by most people. After all, the best alternative sources are the organ meats (liver, kidney, heart, tongue), wheat germ, and yeast. Without milk, therefore, it's not at all easy to get an adequate supply of riboflavin just from food.

Luckily a standard commercial vitamin supplement should supply the riboflavin you need. The RDA is 1.6 milligrams for adult males and 1.2 milligrams for adult females. Pregnant and nursing women should increase that amount to 1.5 and 1.7 milligrams, respectively.

Riboflavin works in your body with enzymes controlling the release of energy from carbohydrates, fats, and proteins. No exotic deficiency disease is associated with the lack of riboflavin, but too little of it can cause a variety of unpleasant symptoms, including lesions found around the mouth and nose, hair loss, and a scaly condition of the skin. It may also contribute to lack of growth in children.

VITAMIN B_{12}

Vitamin B_{12} has a chemical name, cyanocobalamin, but unlike riboflavin, nobody uses it. The *cobal* in the center of its name indicates that the mineral cobalt is a critical part of the vitamin, and so vitamin B_{12} supplies both an essential vitamin and an essential mineral in one package.

Vitamin B_{12} was discovered when doctors were looking for the reason that eating liver cured pernicious anemia, a lack of blood cells that was then always pernicious, or fatal. In fact, vitamin B_{12} is only found in animal foods—liver, kidney, muscle meats, seafood, and eggs. No plants contain it, so vegetarians must supplement their diets with the vitamin.

Extremely tiny doses of the vitamin are all that are necessary. The RDA is only 0.003 milligram for adults, increasing to 0.004 milligram for pregnant and nursing women. Such small doses work because the body carries an enormous store—five or six years' worth—of vitamin B_{12} in the liver. (Other animals do this as well, which is why liver is an excellent source of the vitamin.) Once the stores in the liver are used up, however, much larger doses of vitamin B_{12}—0.015 milligram per day—are required to compensate.

Deficiency symptoms include both blood and nervous system disorders, although pernicious anemia is both rare and curable today. Vitamin B_{12} needs to be combined with calcium during absorption to be properly beneficial, so keeping calcium up to its proper level is essential.

VITAMIN A

Vitamin A is found preformed in animal foods as retinol and in plant foods as carotene, which must be split to form retinol in the body. This is not a very efficient process, but cooking vegetables makes carotene absorption more efficient. Since vitamin A, unlike the B vitamins, is fat soluble, to make use of it, your diet needs to contain an adequate (not excessive) supply of fat.

Carotene is an orange-yellow colored chemical, and orange foods naturally prove to be high in carotene and so in vitamin A. Carrots, pumpkin, squash, apricots, and sweet potatoes are all good sources. Other foods high in vitamin A include liver (of course), and foods whose green color hides their carotene content, like broccoli, spinach, collards, and peppers.

Vitamin A fights infections and aids bone growth and tooth

formation, while a lack of the vitamin causes night blindness. Only extremely tiny doses of the vitamin are needed, which are measured in International Units (IU). Adults need 4000 to 5000 IUs a day, but much higher dosages, up to 100,000 IUs, may be administered for special purposes, like treating acne. Unfortunately, such high doses can be toxic if taken for a long period of time, because vitamin A is stored in the body. Taking any more than the recommended daily dose should be done only under a doctor's care.

NUTRIENTS AND THE LACTOSE INTOLERANT

A sound, nutritious diet is perfectly possible without milk, but calcium is the key. As we've seen, not only is it important in and of itself, but phosphorus, magnesium, and vitamin B_{12} absorption also hinge on an adequate supply of calcium. Calcium supplements are a necessity for virtually everyone who drinks no milk.

Though I've concentrated on the nutrients that are hard to come by without milk in your diet, you can't forget about the others. Whole books have been written on the role of the various nutrients in the diet, so it's not possible for me to cover them here. To give you an idea of which foods are high in which nutrients, turn to Appendix B, which provides a breakdown of the nutrient values of hundreds of foods.

Appendix B can also guide you to those foods that are naturally high in the nutrients you miss if you don't eat milk products. It's possible to go through the book and add up the nutrient content for everything you eat and compare that to the RDA for that nutrient, but that level of work isn't necessary. Make sure you have a good diet, with foods high in the important nutrients, and take calcium supplements. If you do, you'll have no worries about your health even if you never touch another drop of milk.

In the meantime, we need to look at some of the consequences of not having a perfect diet and, more specifically, of not removing lactose from your diet.

WELL-BEING AND YOUR INTESTINES

GAS

At one point in the history of the Roman Empire, laws were passed strictly prohibiting the passing of gas in public places.

Gas may not be illegal today, but it is surely embarrassing and often diabolically uncomfortable. If you have lactose intolerance and you take in too much lactose, you're almost bound to get gas. It's that colony of bacteria in your large intestine busily fermenting the unabsorbed lactose that's at fault. The bacteria produce large amounts of hydrogen, carbon dioxide, and, in some people, methane (all of which are odorless, by the way: nobody knows for sure just what gas actually produces the characteristic smell), leading to bloating, cramps, and heavy flatulence.

Other foods lead to gas as well. Beans have a legendary propensity for gas production, and the legends are well deserved. Beans contain sugars called raffinose and stachyose, which are also fermented by the bacteria in your intestines. Cabbage, cauliflower, and a few fruits (raisins and bananas, as well as apple juice) are other known offenders. The fiber that high-fiber foods are high in is indigestible cellulose, and while this may ease your constipation, those bacteria are at the same time fermenting it and producing gas. Fatty foods and fried foods produce tremendous quantities of carbon dioxide when they hit the natural bicarbonate produced in the intestines. Caffeine, sugar, eggs, beef, chocolate—the list of foods that cause gas or other stomach upsets in some people is endless. If you suspect any one of them, try eliminating it from your diet for a week or so and see how you feel.

Swallowing air is perhaps the major cause of gas among people whose problem doesn't stem from the foods they eat. Many people swallow air all day long as a nervous habit, without even noticing that they do so. Even for those without this habit, the simple act of swallowing food puts air into your stomach. Gassy drinks, like beer and soda pop, are obvious sources of air in food, but air is also whipped into bread and ice cream. Even an apple may contain 20 percent air.

Eliminating the gas associated with lactose intolerance is as straightforward as switching to a lactose-free diet. If that isn't enough, then stay away from other gassy foods and be careful not to swallow air as a habit.

Still not enough? Many people try taking antacids for relief. If your problem is lactose intolerance, then antacids will not help: they work entirely in the stomach, while the gas produced by bacteria is hidden far away in your intestines. Nothing will neutralize intestinal gas. All you can do is try to work it out of your body.

As I pointed out in Chapter 2, our bodies were designed by millions of years of creation to work best in certain ways that a few thousand years of civilization have not changed. Primitive humans defecated in a squatting position, with their thighs pushed up against their stomachs. Squatting not only helps gas but may also release the feces trapped by gas bubbles in the intestines, useful in times of mild constipation and when the gas is trapping loose diarrhea inside.

Another way of expelling gas was suggested to me to relieve the horrendous gas pains that can be produced by a barium enema, although the technique is also useful at other times. Gas will sometimes get caught in the kinks in the intestines. Lying on your stomach and slowly and gently rolling onto your side, onto your back, onto your other side, and back again to your stomach allows gravity to pull at the gas, much like tilting a marble in a hand-held maze helps it roll toward the goal.

In a more public setting, find a hard straight chair to sit in. Fold your arms across your middle and apply gentle pressure. If the gas is creating pain in one spot, use one hand to massage that area.

Along with these do's are a couple of don'ts. Don't lie down immediately after a meal. The change in the positioning of your stomach may decrease burping but will increase flatulence. A leisurely walk is much better medicine. Also, don't strain at gas to try to expel it. Straining at gas and stool may lead to hemorrhoids. Instead, try to relax your body and muscles as much as possible. Stress and strain of any kind are bad for your intestines.

Relaxation allows the body to do what it does naturally—pass a cup to a quart of gas each day, whether we know it or not.

DIARRHEA

If you get diarrhea because of lactose intolerance, there is one safe, sure, and effective cure: stop eating foods that contain lactose. At the very least, reduce the quantity of lactose so that it's low enough to stop causing diarrhea as a symptom.

Diarrhea in adults is mostly an annoyance, but in children, the loss of body fluids and electrolytes—salts that are required to maintain chemical balances in the body—can be dangerous. Infalyte and Pedialyte are solutions that provide both needed fluid and the chemicals being lost. Both are available without a prescription.

You can provide the same benefits at home by preparing these mixtures recommended by the Federal Centers for Disease Control. Glass 1: add ½ teaspoon of honey or corn syrup and a pinch of table salt to 8 ounces of orange, apple, or other fruit juice. Glass 2: add ½ teaspoon of baking soda to 8 ounces of water. Drink alternately from each glass. Repeat throughout the day. Adults and children can drink other beverages in between but should stay away from solid foods. Infants should continue breast-feeding and drink plain water while also receiving these salt solutions. Long-term diarrhea in an infant is serious and may be a sign of lactose intolerance or other dietary problems. If the diarrhea persists, see your pediatrician.

The Food and Drug Administration has convened a series of Advisory Review Panels on over-the-counter (OTC) medications during the past several years. A few medications have been deemed safe and effective for the treatment of diarrhea by the FDA's Advisory Panel on OTC Miscellaneous Internal Drug Products. One is diphenoxylate hydrochloride, which is sold under many brand names, including Lotomil, Loflo, L-Trol, and Colonaid. Diphenoxylate relaxes the colon, reducing cramps, and allows more water to be absorbed. It is also an opiate, so it is likely to be available by prescription only, at least in effective doses.

The other safe and effective drug is polycarbophil, sold under the brand name Mitrolan. Polycarbophil absorbs sixty times its weight in water and so allows the stool to solidify. It's the only over-the-counter diarrhea medication approved for young children.

None of the other numerous brands of antidiarrhea medicines has been found safe and effective, because of either unsafe ingredients, ingredients without proved effectiveness, or too-small doses of those ingredients that seem to work.

Rather than relying on these drugs, you'd be much better off to change your diet or that of your child and remove those foods that cause the diarrhea in the first place.

HEMORRHOIDS

Hemorrhoids bear an uncomfortable similarity to lactose intolerance. They're both associated with aging, and they're both far more common than most people suspect. More than half the adults in this country have hemorrhoids, although (and again the similarity to lactose intolerance) the symptoms may be so mild that they aren't even aware that anything is wrong.

Hemorrhoids are blood vessels from the anus that engorge with blood when you put pressure on them, as happens when you strain to push things out. When you're younger, these veins shrink again when the pressure is released, but as you grow older, this no longer happens as easily. They may push out of the anus and be trapped by the muscle of the anal sphincter. Hemorrhoids, therefore, can be either internal or external; both will bleed, but the external ones usually cause the most pain.

Diarrhea sufferers, especially older adults, know that a bout of diarrhea that lasts more than a day or two will often result in hemorrhoids. But constipation will do the same thing if force is used to try to expel the trapped stool. Pregnant women may notice hemorrhoids forming as early in their pregnancy as their morning sickness. (While truck drivers are the subject of many hemorrhoid jokes, the truth is that people who sit all day long get no more hemorrhoids than do those who are physically active. Both baseball player George Brett and Jimmy Carter while President suffered through well-publicized hemorrhoid episodes.)

Severe hemorrhoids can be removed by surgery in several

ways, in operations ranging in seriousness from a minor doctor's office visit to a major surgical production called a hemorrhoid-ectomy. Before you allow matters to get that serious, you can—and should—do several things yourself.

First, keep the area clean. Be gentle, pat rather than rub, and use soft toilet tissue or tissue moistened with water on the tender area. Use baby powder afterward to keep the region dry. To relieve the swelling, the best and cheapest cure is a sitz bath. Special bowls are made for hemorrhoid sufferers to sit in, but running water into your bathtub will do just fine. Doctors disagree about how hot the water should be—some say warm and some say very hot—but all agree that a fifteen-to-thirty minute sitz bath two to four times a day is the best medicine.

Doctors also disagree about the effectiveness of medications such as Preparation H, which is by far the leading over-the-counter medication in the hemorrhoid field. Even the ones who do recommend its use say it should only be used for occasional relief of symptoms and should by no means be thought of as a cure. According to the FDA panel on hemorrhoids, a medication that will do the same job as Preparation H at a much lower cost is plain petroleum jelly. Petroleum jelly protects the region against further irritation and relieves pain, burning, and itching.

More agreement is reached about the need for a high-fiber diet, since the fiber helps soften the stool and make it easier to remove.

One thing everyone insists upon is that if you bleed from the anus, you must go see a doctor. Although the odds are extremely good that nothing worse than hemorrhoids is wrong with you, blood from the anus is also a sign of colon cancer, which should absolutely be caught as early as possible.

WARNING! THIS PILL CONTAINS LACTOSE

After you've read every food label in the supermarket, after you've purged your shelves of every box, bag, and can inhabited by a milk product, after you've bought every milk substitute you've ever heard of, you're still not completely safe. You may be swallowing lactose every time you place a pill in your mouth.

Pills in tablet form are often made by placing the medicines in machines that punch the ingredients together. Lactose, because it absorbs water, acts as a binder and holds the whole pill together. The mildly sweet lactose powder is also useful for bulking out the powder in capsules, so that no air spaces are left. Shiny coatings on pills can be lactose, and in some time-release capsules, those tiny time pellets inside are each and every one lactose coated. By one estimate, lactose is used in 20 percent of all prescription drugs. Since some prescription drugs are in liquid form, unlikely to contain lactose, the percentage of lactose-containing tablets and capsules must be even higher.

Now, if 20 percent of prescription drugs have lactose, that means that 80 percent do not. Fewer nonprescription (over-the-counter) medications contain lactose than those that are lactose free. And in general, the amount of lactose in prescription and over-the-counter drugs is small. Small doesn't mean insignificant, but it's impossible to pack as much lactose into a tiny pill as you would get from a glass of milk. The big problem comes when lactose shows up in the wrong place. For example, Milicon, an antigas tablet often recommended by doctors to ease gas pains, contains lactose in each chewable tablet. (Liquid Milicon is lactose free, however, like most liquids.) Chewing these pills all day long could give severely lactose-intolerant people more gas than when they started. In fact, the reason studies of Milicon's active ingredient, simethicone, have been so inconclusive may be that the lactose was causing gas at the same time the simethicone was trying to relieve it.

Milicon may have as much as one-third of a gram of lactose in each tablet. Other pills, especially when the lactose is used only as a coating, will have much less lactose. Unless you are unusually sensitive, you would have to abuse most medications before the lactose caused symptoms, just as most people can drink some milk with no problems whatsoever. And yet people say, both to doctors and to the drug companies, that they feel better because they've stopped taking pills containing lactose.

If you wanted to check whether your medication has lactose in it, how would you do so? Through 1985, there was no way short of writing to the manufacturer and asking. In 1985, however, a major consumer victory was won. Three associations of drug manufacturers—the Pharmaceutical Manufacturers Association, whose members make most of the prescription drugs in the country; the Generic Pharmaceutical Industry Association, composed of major independent distributors of generic prescription drugs; and the Proprietary Association, manufacturers of most of the over-the-counter, nonprescription medications—have all agreed on a series of voluntary standards to disclose inactive ingredients. Inactive ingredients include fillers, binders, disintegrating agents, coatings, colors, and flavors. By the time you read this book, unless a package has been sitting on a store shelf since 1985, all the medicines you see (except for a very few from small companies that are not members of the three associations) will be accompanied by a full list of inactive ingredients along with the active ones.

The different kinds of medicines are treated in different ways. Over-the-counter medications have the list of inactive ingredients printed right on the box, much like the ingredient lists on food packages. If lactose is an ingredient, you'll see it listed there, by name.

Since prescription drugs don't come in neat little boxes suitable for labeling, the ingredients lists are included on the official package insert that contains the other information doctors use in deciding whether a medication is appropriate for you. (Samples and drugs destined for institutions rather than pharmacies also should have ingredients lists included, according to the guidelines.) You should be able to ask your doctor to see this, or you could get the same information from the *Physicians Desk Reference*, a standard reference book that virtually all doctors—and public libraries—get. Pharmacists will also have access to this type of information. Your doctor should know you have lactose intolerance (if not, tell him or her *right away*) and will be able to check for lactose content before prescribing a drug.

Remember, these guidelines are voluntary, not mandated by any governmental agency. Although there's no reason to believe that the manufacturers won't go along with them, only time will tell. Since the guidelines are voluntary, there are no penalties for not complying. Only the thought of what consumers and consumer groups might say or do will keep the manufacturers honest. Another problem with voluntary guidelines is that they can be changed at will, without anyone going through the bother of issuing a press release to let the public know.

Another, more immediate problem with the guidelines is that they are really set up more to warn people about substances to which they may be allergic. In an allergy, the amount of the substance present doesn't matter that much. All anyone cares about is whether that ingredient is present or absent. For this reason, the guidelines merely state that the manufacturers have to list all the inactive ingredients in alphabetical order, not in order by amount. Lactose intolerance gets worse the more lactose is present, but the current guidelines give you no way of knowing whether that is a great deal or a very small amount. The best guidelines of all from a consumer standpoint would have all manufacturers (of both food and drugs) list not only every ingredient but also the quantity of every ingredient. That's something to fight for in the future.

Manufacturers also do not have to list an ingredient if its presence is a trade secret (although some of the guidelines tighten this loophole slightly). Lactose is unlikely to be a trade secret, but those of you allergic to other substances may find that full disclosure would have been much better for you.

Although the guidelines aren't perfect, the possibility of having this much-needed information available is exciting. In the past, doctors prescribing certain medications sometimes had to discontinue their use because of the side effects they caused. Stomach or intestinal operations, for example, can cause secondary or acquired lactose intolerance. But the antibiotic capsules used to fight infections after the operation may themselves have lactose. Result: agonizing gas cramps. Doctors, not realizing that lactose was the problem, would assume the antibiotic was causing the reaction and so would replace it with a second choice, one possibly more toxic or expensive. With the new labeling guidelines, doctors can pick and choose from all the antibiotics to get one that is effective and lactose free the first time around.

You can do the same when looking for over-the-counter medications. If there is no good substitute, I wouldn't pass up any helpful medication just because of a small dose of lactose; curing whatever is wrong with you is worth taking the small chance of getting symptoms from the lactose. But if there are two equally good drugs, and one contains lactose and the other doesn't, by all means go for the lactose-free one. You'll be doing your body a favor and striking another blow for smart consumerism.

CHAPTER ELEVEN

EATING OUT IN COMFORT AND SAFETY

MILK-FREE HOMES AWAY FROM HOME

Some of my friends and relatives simply stopped inviting me for dinner after they learned I had lactose intolerance. Others tried going to great lengths to prepare meals they thought I could eat, without checking with me first. I still remember the occasion I had a forkful of beef bourguignon to my lips while my hostess bragged that she had used substitutes for everything, in fact, had even used margarine instead of butter because margarine never had any milk. I gently informed her about the facts of nondairy life.

Before you drive all your friends paranoid or, worse, away, take a minute to decide how fanatic on the subject of lactose you need to be. If you're only mildly intolerant, you can probably survive a single meal at an outsider's house with no great discomfort, no matter what is served, especially if you take some lactase pills along with the meal. Silence is golden and almost certainly beats trying to explain to your elderly aunt Mildred why she has to alter her cherished recipe for creamed eggplant that was the hit of the last five family reunions.

Those of us with more severe intolerance don't have much choice; it's either explain the situation or not eat. Given a choice like that, I'll explain every time. (Of course, it doesn't hurt to remember that some hosts like to fuss. Give them an excuse to go out of their way to provide you with a proper meal, and they feel happily martyred for the whole dinner. Cultivate these people.)

How much information you give them depends upon the situation in which you find yourself. Overkill isn't necessary. I'd like it if you bought everyone at whose house you ever planned to eat a copy of this book with orders to read it, but that's going a bit far. Remember, you're trying to allay their fears of upsetting you as much as you're trying to protect yourself.

First of all, make sure that they know what lactose intolerance is and what the problem ingredients might be. Like my relative I just mentioned, most people think that all margarine is milk free, not just a few selected brands. At the same time (probably because eggs are so often classified as dairy foods), most people have the mistaken idea that mayonnaise is forbidden. Here's where the time you've spent studying recipes in cookbooks and searching the supermarket aisles for lactose-free products proves its worth. You'll know as soon as you hear the menu for the planned meal where the real trouble spots might be and be able to suggest alterations or substitutions to get both you and your hosts off the hook. Result: grateful hosts and a worry-free meal.

Keeping the suggestions simple is the important part. After all, you can't transform somebody else's kitchen on your behalf. Explain about milk-free margarine and Coffee Rich, and how easily they substitute for butter and cream. Suggest oil and vinegar or a brand of milk-free salad dressing for the salad. Recommend that the cheese sauce be poured over everyone else's individual serving rather than over the entire dish. Offer to buy a loaf of french bread to complement the meal. Suggest fruit for dessert rather than cheesecake, or one of the tofu "ice creams" rather than the real thing. You don't want your hosts to feel harried and guilty, and you don't want to fret over every bite. Keep it light and simple and you'll be invited back.

One thing you can do to help out is bring along your own

supplies (to use at the table or to drop off beforehand) rather than make your hosts buy milk substitutes they'll never use again. Miss Manners may not approve of the custom, but I find that it's reassuring all around.

Overnight stays are another problem that can be solved by a little judicious shopping on your own. The one-time-only nature of dinners makes them easier to handle than a several-day visit, especially since breakfasts without milk are harder to fake. When I spent a week at a friend's house recently, I brought along a cache of bagels from my favorite bakery, bought some margarine at a local supermarket, found little containers of a milk substitute at a convenience store, and had breakfast supplies for my whole stay. For dinners (after a first night's repast of a cheeseless spaghetti sauce), we went out to restaurants. This made life easier on my hosts by shifting the entire burden to me, a burden I'm happy to accept.

THE SUBTLE ART OF EATING OUT

One-third of all American meals are eaten in restaurants. Every day's newspaper reports another new restaurant opening: gourmet dining, fast-food emporiums, ethnic specialties of every description, dessert palaces where the calories are calibrated in thousands. No reason in the world you should feel locked out of these places just because you have lactose intolerance. All you need is a strategy to deal with unfamiliar menus.

Once again, these comments are aimed at those with severe lactose intolerance, who truly want to avoid all milk if it is at all possible. The rest of you should be able to get through a meal safely virtually anywhere as long as you don't overwhelm your system with glorious and exotic dishes overflowing with butter and cheese and cream. Always carry a supply of lactase pills with you, and don't be afraid to take as many as necessary. Then eat and enjoy.

Cuisines Without Milk

With most of the cultures in the world filled with lactose-intolerant people, it shouldn't surprise you that their cuisines are largely milk free. The authentic cuisines, that is. Trouble is, so many ethnic dishes have been adapted to American tastes (or even invented by Americans) that milk has crept in along the edges almost everywhere.

Kosher Restaurants

If you want an absolute, certified guarantee that you will get no milk products of any description, the only place to go is a true kosher restaurant. (These restaurants, sometimes called *glatt* kosher, should not be confused with "Kosher-style" restaurants, where no safety is guaranteed.) As I explained in Chapter 8, the kosher dietary laws require that meat and milk never be mixed, so if you order any meat dish, you will not be served anything else that contains milk, even if you ask for it. You'll automatically get milk-free margarine for your milk-free bread and rolls and a milk substitute for your coffee. Reuben sandwiches will come without the cheese and potatoes without any sour cream.

One thing you'd better remember is that this separation doesn't mean there are no milk products on the premises. Dairy products can be perfectly kosher, as long as they are served without meat. You can get sour cream for your potatoes if you order them with, say, fish, and cheesecake is a grand old deli specialty. And what good would a deli be if you couldn't get bagels with lox and cream cheese? To avoid getting any of these, just say that other magic Jewish word, *pareve*. Pareve foods are neutral, neither milk nor meat, and so can be eaten with either. Sticking with meat and pareve foods is a guarantee that you can leave your lactase pills home and never trouble your head about what you eat.

Kosher restaurants, even when they're more than delis, tend to have solid meat-and-potato type hearty, heavy foods. If you're looking for something lighter that can also be a bit more elegant, the next safest variety of restaurants is Asian.

Asian Restaurants

A few years ago, all Asian restaurants were Chinese, but today you can easily find Japanese, Thai, Vietnamese, Indonesian, and Korean restaurants in all large cities and most medium-size ones. Asian restaurants come in all degrees of elegance, from the equivalent of greasy spoons to overpriced palaces, but all aside from the cheapest place a premium on meticulously cooked and aesthetically arranged food.

Chinese restaurants are everywhere, even in cities without a Chinatown. For many years, Chinese cooking meant Cantonese-style, with the dishes at the lower end of scale—chow mein and chop suey—unknown in China, invented instead by Chinese cooks in the old West. Recently, with the barriers to China coming down, various Chinese regional cuisines have become more widely available. Szechwan-, Hunan-, Mandarin-, Peking-, and Shanghai-style dishes are common on Chinese restaurant menus today. No one chef is likely to be equally good at all of these (just as no cook would be at home simultaneously with French, German, Italian, and Irish cookery), but barring the occasional piece of exotica like fresh fried milk with crabmeat, the only danger of coming into contact with a milk product in a Chinese restaurant is in the ice cream or sherbet that is the usual dessert.

The newer Asian cuisines vary tremendously in scope and style. Japanese steak houses are now being challenged by restaurants serving sushi and sashimi, featuring the raw fish and seaweed Americans are just beginning to learn to appreciate. Both are likely to serve shrimp or other foods done tempura-style, or fried in a light batter. Tempura batter is usually milk free; if you have any doubts, be sure to ask.

Now that American palates have been warmed by the spiciness of Szechwan and Hunan cuisines, the even hotter foods from other Far Eastern countries are making their appearance. Thai food is rumored to be among the hottest in the world; Koreans make much use of chili peppers; and Indonesian dishes can be fiery to the unwary. None ordinarily uses much milk in the preparation, although chefs do make efforts to adapt to American tastes and American foods.

Indian food is much more of a problem. Cows are a fixture in India to an extent unknown further east, so milk is as much a part of the basic diet as it is in western Europe. *Kheer* is rice cooked in milk; *dal* is a creamy lentil side dish; *kofta* are meatballs made with a cream sauce. Some dishes, such as the lamb-based *roghan josh*, are cooked in a yogurt rather a cream sauce. Yogurt is far better tolerated than milk and cream by most people who are lactose intolerant, so you may decide to chance such foods. Stay away from the desserts, though, unless you know exactly what is in them. Most Indian desserts are heavy on the milk products.

All-American Cuisine

Thousands of other ethnic restaurants dot the highways and side streets of America, with the larger cities boasting varieties unknown elsewhere. Ethiopian restaurants may well serve a milk-free menu, but that knowledge does hardly anyone outside of Washington and New York any good.

But while you're out exploring out-of-the-way restaurants (preferably with a good native guide), let me remind you of one other type of ethnic restaurant so common you may not even think of it as such: the all-American steak house.

A few of the more elegant restaurants may sauté steaks in butter, but the traditional charcoal-broiled steak (found in Argentinian restaurants, too, by the way) never gets close to a milk product once it leaves the cow. Charcoal-broiled anything, from seafood to hamburger, is among the safest bets to order in a restaurant, though you should stick to milk-free breads rather than rolls when ordering hamburgers. Especially beware of the places that carefully brush your hamburger roll with butter before serving it to you brown and toasted.

In less adventurous cities, restaurateurs learn quickly that while coquilles Saint-Jacques and veal Orloff may make a few customers and the chefs happy, a large-size prime rib on the menu is necessary to make a profit and keep the chefs paid. It's just as well. We can't eat the other dishes, but prime rib is almost always safe. Steak and prime rib don't make for adventurous

dining, but they have the virtue of being found almost everywhere.

Making Meals Milk-Proof

So you've been invited to join the crowd for dinner, and your
frantic suggestion to go Chinese has been ignored. Not to worry.
Unless you're going to a French restaurant so haute cuisine that
even the menu is in French, you should be able to pilot your way
to a milk-free evening without being forced to fall back upon the
tiresome standby of a slab of rare or well-done meat.

If you begin meals with a drink, you probably know that Irish
cream whiskeys, Häagen-Dazs liqueur, and similar spirits are
trendy additions to a bewildering variety of new drinks. These
liqueurs boast real cream among their ingredients, placing drinks
made with them on the taboo list. As with almost every other
food, there is a milk-free substitute. The whiskeys that spell their
names "creme" are nondairy equivalents. If you don't know for
sure what a drink contains, ask. It definitely won't be the last
time you do during that evening.

The real work of the meal starts when the menu arrives. First
scan the menu for any friendly, familiar dishes you know to be
both safe and delicious. If nothing surfaces, read over the entire
menu very carefully. Rather than sticking to traditional entrées,
you may decide to build a meal out of milk-free items from among
the soups, appetizers, and salads. Approach the menu as a creative
opportunity rather than a rigidly segmented straitjacket.

Assuming you're having a more traditional evening out, you'll
look first at the appetizers and soups. Unfortunately these vary
so tremendously that few rules can be laid out. The ubiquitous
shrimp cocktail is one food almost sure to be safe, however, as
are most clear (i.e., not creamy) soups.

Once past the opening courses, examine the entrées carefully.
Don't expect to learn much from their names alone. While some
are standardized by tradition, too many others are fanciful nonsense (possibly invented by a professional menu writer) or are
of the chicken à la Alphonse variety, paying pretentious homage

to the owner's name. Lately, though, I've noticed more and more restaurants attempting to attract new customers and save staff time on explanations (not to mention making the food sound better) by lavishly describing the contents of each entrée.

Sauces are almost bound to be your downfall. Many foods just aren't considered complete without a sauce, and most of the sauces in the world contain butter or cream. The French are notorious for the richness of their sauces. Béarnaise, béchamel, hollandaise, mornay, and soubise sauces in the classic tradition include milk in one form or another as a basic ingredient. Bordelaise and lyonnaise sauces don't call for butter directly, but Escoffier directs that the shallots or onions they do contain be cooked in butter before being added. This milk at one remove rather reduces the amount of lactose that could be present (since butter is so low in lactose in the first place), but it points up the necessity of a thorough knowledge of food if you want to completely rid yourself of lactose while dining chicly.

The Italians offer you a better chance at milk-free sauces than the French, but you can still expect carbonara, alfredo, and pesto sauces to be on the forbidden list. Assume, too, that any basic spaghetti sauce will contain cheese. While chefs' recipes are highly individualistic, bolognese, marinara, or primavera sauces are better choices for a milk-free alternative. Orange sauces, as in duck à la orange, create another opportunity for slipping around the milk-laden dishes.

Never forget that your chef may use secret recipes that alter the ingredients entirely, increasing the thrill of the risk. Will asking the chef help? Not necessarily. In large restaurants, sauces are composed by the daytime chefs. Whoever is in the kitchen in the evening, however great a chef, may have no firm idea of what went into them.

Cheeses are a dead giveaway, of course, and cheese sauces are found on hundreds of otherwise appetizing dishes. Most of these meals depend upon the cheese for flavor, so asking for them without the cheese almost guarantees a bland and tasteless dinner, assuming it is within the dignity of the chef to make it at all.

Sautés are another problem. All the better restaurants use naught but butter for sautéing, while lesser ones still rely on liquid margarine or an oil-butter mixture. Similarly, foods that are broiled (not charcoal-broiled), especially fish, are often dotted with butter to help moisten them and bring out their flavor. Meals made this way must be made to order, however, which gives you the opportunity to custom-make your dish. It is no great imposition for the chef to substitute a vegetable oil for the butter while sautéing or to use lemon juice when oven-broiling fish. You should realize that the fish tends to come out a bit drier this way—too dry if not watched very carefully.

Fried foods, or any foods that come in a breading or encased in dough, are also to be avoided. Not only are the bread crumbs likely to have been made with milk, but some fried foods are dipped in milk before being breaded. Beef or any of the other Wellingtons are made by encasing the meat in pastry loaded with butter. Croissants, so popular and common that even Burger King leads its breakfast menu with them, drip butter. Milk-free croissants are as imaginary as the Loch Ness monster.

Once you've narrowed the entrées to a short list that sounds both good and milk free, it's time to talk to the waiter or waitress. Don't assume that they'll know the ingredients of all the dishes on the menu. Odds are good that their knowledge barely exceeds yours. Good chefs don't go spreading their recipes around.

Explain your problem simply but exactly. Do not say you have lactose intolerance, which will get you no more than a polite smile and a blank look. Comprehension improves if you make it clear that you have to avoid milk products and then specifically mention the ones most likely to be used in preparing the food (milk, cream, cheese, butter). Ask the waiter or waitress to ask the chef if any of those milk products are in the dishes you are considering. If you've sorted through the menu well, at least one of your choices should be okay. Rarely, every dish will number milk products among its ingredients. If that occurs, fall upon the mercy of the restaurant by asking that the chef recommend a milk-free entrée. Be prepared to wind up with a dish that would have been twenty-third on your list if you had free power of choice.

Even with the entrée settled, many more questions need to be asked and choices made. You can assume the rolls brought to the table have been made with milk. Again, asking the help may do little good; in many restaurants, the dough is shipped in frozen or as a mix from a wholesale distributor. (If I suspect this, I'll add whey to the list of milk products I say I can't have, since the packages for the rolls may include a list of ingredients whey may be one of.) A tip: frozen dough, when finished baking, often gets brushed with butter to simulate a fresh-baked appearance. French or Italian breads are nice safe alternatives. In fact, if the restaurant is open for lunch, some of those breads or rye or pumpernickel may be leftover sandwich material, which the waiter or waitress is usually happy to bring out specially for you.

When ordering a salad, always remember to specify that they leave out the croutons. Salad dressings, while fraught with traps, still leave plenty of milk-free opportunities. Virtually every restaurant will serve oil and vinegar (or vinaigrette, sometimes with added spices or mustard). French, Italian, Russian, and Thousand Island dressings are usually okay if made with mayonnaise and no cream. Ask your waiter or waitress to double-check if you want to be sure, especially if any of the dressings are labeled creamy. (Ranch and bleu cheese dressings are out everywhere.) Cole slaw or potato and macaroni salads are safe everywhere, except in a restaurant I ate in while writing this chapter, where the cole slaw arrived in a dressing mixed with sour cream (as was the Russian dressing). No generalization is absolute in cookery, but by knowing the right questions to ask, you can save yourself endless problems.

Vegetables have two major styles: cooked in butter or steamed. You want the steamed, of course. Rarely can you get the chef to steam vegetables just for you. With a microwave in every restaurant nowadays, you can ask that the vegetables be microwaved plain with a bit of liquid, a procedure much easier on the chef. Baked potatoes and french fries are milk free, if you remember to specify that you want no butter or sour cream on the baked potato. Mashed, scalloped, au gratin, and princess potatoes, on the other hand, come loaded with milk products. Also beware of baked stuffed potatoes, since the stuffing is seldom anything you can eat. Rice is so often made with butter that you'll have few chances to eat it in any but Asian restaurants.

Desserts in restaurants are for wistfully sighing over rather than for eating. Everything that looks good—from cakes to pies to tortes to sundaes—is loaded with lactose. Fruit dishes are a nice alternative, especially in summer, when chilled fruit tops off a meal lightly and pleasantly. Of course, you can stick to plain coffee and tea, giving yourself something to do while everyone else finishes dessert. (You'd better like your coffee black, since the odds are vanishingly small that you'll find a nondairy creamer in a better restaurant.) On the other hand, having nothing at all can make your companions feel so guilty that they pick up the check in sheer embarrassment. My friends have learned better, but you may have innocent victims to try this game on.

When the check does come, assuming that you're paying your share, there's always the question of what to tip the waiter or waitress. Special requests are not so unusual that you should feel obligated to tip big just because he or she made an extra trip to ask the chef a question. However, special attention and handling deserve to be rewarded. A waiter or waitress who takes the trouble to ask about items on the menu without any prompting, or suggests milk-free alternatives, or offers a substitution I would not have known about otherwise always gets a good-size tip at the end of the meal because the evening has been made that much more enjoyable.

One final suggestion for restaurant dining: Become a regular patron at a particular restaurant with a good menu and plenty of milk-free side dishes. Restaurant owners naturally try a little harder to please their regular customers, so you won't be locked into the menu. Actually many restaurants will prepare special meals if arrangements are made at least a day in advance. Realistically, though, you stand a better chance of getting accommodated if the owner knows your name and the help have seen you throw something extra into the tip each time you dine there. You should also follow through on the standards of restaurant etiquette—make reservations each time you dine, even if the restaurant is not likely to be crowded (for one thing, this makes sure the owner knows your name), and always arrive on time.

Restaurant dining will never be as safe as eating in your own milk-proofed house. Avoiding restaurants, however, turns lactose intolerance from an inconvenience into a handicap. Few people can eat everything everywhere—few would even want to. You may be restricted in your preferences, but the vast majority of restaurants are open to you, and you should always be able to find something on the menu that's right for you.

FAST FOOD, OR WHERE TO EAT ON THE INTERSTATE

Beating up on fast food is a favorite sport among food critics. Fast food has been accused of being cheap, plastic, less tasty than the containers it comes in, and destructive of the individuality of American cooking. Most of this is nonsense, especially the latter. I'd rather eat in a spotlessly clean fast-food outlet than in most of the greasy-spoon restaurants put out of business by the rise of the franchises. Besides, with the tens of thousands of franchised food emporiums in the country, they're a cultural phenomenon. Kids love them, adults appreciate their convenience, and only a few curmudgeons stay away entirely.

Most of all, fast food has played upon the rootlessness and desire for security of mobile American culture. Rather than playing the age-old guessing game of choosing a decent restaurant while on the road, the traveling family chooses the quick, easy, and reliable way out: a familiar name far from home. The big name chains know this and take advantage of it. As Burger Kings replace more traditional restaurants at the rest stops on the New York Thruway, you'll have to drive miles out of your way to avoid them.

Given all this, I wish I had better news for you about eating fast food. The lactose intolerant can find fast food to eat, but not with much choice. None of my good advice for better restaurants applies to fast-food places. Menus are smaller and more restrictive, side dishes are limited, special arrangements run more toward taking a pickle off a bun than finding a substitute for the bun itself. The help in the major franchised operations often don't even know what the ingredients in the food are: buns come out of faraway regional distributors, while batters are prepared from premixed batches.

I tried writing to the major nationwide chains asking for milk-free foods we could eat and received very little response. On the grounds that what you don't know can hurt you, I'd be very careful when entering any fast-food outlet.

McDonald's

Now for the good news. The classic among classics when it comes to fast food is the McDonald's basic meal of a burger, fries, and soft drink, the meal that a 50-billion-plus empire was built upon. And it is all lactose free. You could even have a Big Mac, as long as you ordered it without the cheese. I don't know what else is in the secret sauce, but milk is not one of the ingredients.

Not much else at McDonald's is lactose free, I'm sorry to say. The following long list was supplied to me by McDonald's; everything in it contains lactose.

hotcakes	hot chocolate	English muffins
hot fudge	sundae mix	Chicken McNuggets
biscuits	danish pastries	eggs fried in butter
caramel	milk shake mix	chocolate chip cookies
cheese	birthday cake	
pies		

The hamburgers are all beef, the buns are milk free everywhere in the United States, and the french fries use dextrose instead of lactose for browning. That adds up to a meal—admittedly a limited one, but one that millions have enjoyed.

Domino's Pizza and Pizza Hut

Ever tried a cheeseless pizza? Pizza is not pizza without cheese, but what's left can be surprisingly tasty. Unfortunately, the same warning I gave about spaghetti sauce applies to pizza sauce as well: assume it contains cheese unless assured otherwise.

Whether that means you avoid pizza is up to you. Cheese is rather low in lactose to begin with, and the amounts used in most sauces aren't necessarily high. Domino's Pizza chain, for example, uses a sauce containing one-half of one percent (that's 1 part in 200) of Romano cheese. At Pizza Hut, both the pizza sauce and the pan pizza crust contain milk products. If you tell the cook to leave off the Cheddar cheese, then their Taco Pizza on either the Thin 'N Crispy or Thick 'N Chewy crusts will be milk free.

Pizza Hut has a much wider menu selection than straight pizza places, giving you other foods to consider. There is no cheese in either their meat or meatless pasta sauces. Order them with the spaghetti, but skip the meatballs, because the meatballs do contain cheese. They even say that the garlic bread is safe if you specify that the seasoning cheese be left off. A trip to the salad bar will make a nice accompaniment, but watch out for the Romano, Blue Cheese, Lite Cucumber, and Hidden Valley Ranch® salad dressings, as well as the croutons. Bread for sandwiches is purchased locally by the restaurants, so you'll have to ask and see if anyone there can find an ingredients list.

Baskin-Robbins Ice Cream

The people at Baskin-Robbins answered my query and sent me an ad for Chocolate month at the same time, leaving me with very mixed feelings. However, while all the chocolate ice creams (and every other) contain milk products, the Baskin-Robbins ices (no chocolate, alas) and their raspberry sorbet do not.

Orange Julius

That mysterious powder that gives the various flavors of Julius beverages at an Orange Julius that distinct flavor and texture contains whole milk powder. All the other products in the stores (hot dogs, sandwiches, etc.) are made from ingredients purchased locally. Your best bet would be to contact the manager of your nearest Orange Julius and see if he or she can dig up ingredients lists for those.

Kentucky Fried Chicken

One of the Big Secrets in William Poundstone's book of the same name is the secret behind Kentucky Fried Chicken batter. The secret herbs and spices may still be in dispute, but Poundstone quotes from the patent filed by Col. Harlan Sanders for the fried chicken that was the basis of his coast-to-coast chain. The patent reads that the chicken pieces are "immersed in a dip made of skimmed or reconstituted skimmed milk..."

I received no answer from Kentucky Fried Chicken when trying to confirm this, but this method of making chicken is so common that I would stay away from most fried chicken places just to be safe.

With hundreds of fast-food chains in America, and few of them truly nationwide, I can't be of too much help in pointing out the milk-free dishes. Again, my advice is to ask the manager to list the foods without milk, but don't be surprised if you don't get a very good answer. If you can find an address for the chain headquarters, try writing. You may have better luck than I did.

Traveling Without Milk

All the long hard hours of work you put in to free your life of lactose vanish once you travel away from home, even if you travel only within the United States. The brands in the supermarket change, the local bakeries are unknowns, restaurants display unfamiliar menus with regional dishes you've never heard of, and the refrigerator stocked with milk-free substitutes is miles from your hotel room.

Nevertheless, European visitors are often amazed (or dismayed) at how similar one American city is to any other. You can make these broad similarities work for you to overcome individual differences as you travel. The names may change, but the basic principles underlying a lactose-free diet will work no matter where you go.

If you've grown used to national brands of milk-free foods (or even store brands sold in nationwide chains), you'll find them virtually everywhere in the country. For many items, however, I have to rely on regional or local brands, which cater to less middle-of-the-road tastes than the national brands do. Since I seldom see these lesser-known brands outside my local stores, my only alternative while away from home is to spend even more time reading ingredients lists up and down store aisles until I can find substitutes.

Basics, like Coffee Rich, Mocha Mix on the West Coast, or house-brand milk substitutes and milk-free margarine, are easy to find anywhere. Good breads may take more searching. Check the local phone directory for any Jewish bakeries in the area, and patronize them for their pareve breads and rolls. Italian bakeries are sources of Italian bread, usually milk free, and rolls and other items made from the same dough.

This all assumes you have time to shop and a refrigerator to put the food in. If you take the hotel route, you may eat in restaurants three times a day. Here, again, apply what you've learned from eating out in your hometown. Use the phone book, travel or restaurant guides, or the local newspaper to learn about the restaurants available. (If you're lucky, you may have friends who know the area and can guide you.) By being adventurous at home, you should have built up a repertoire of types of restaurants and dishes you like.

Once you're in a likely sounding restaurant, behave exactly as you would at any new restaurant at home, being doubly careful to study the menu and quiz the help about the contents of the dishes.

Breakfasts are especially troublesome while traveling, since so many of the common breakfast foods either contain milk products (cereal with milk, toast and butter, pancakes) or are usually cooked in butter (eggs, sausages). If you can get the chef to use a vegetable oil when cooking your food, you may be safe, but I can't guarantee you much success.

One trick I've learned is that a stick of milk-free margarine (or at least part of one) will fit nicely into a wide-mouth vacuum bottle, along with two or three restaurant-size single-serving containers of Coffee Rich. Packed with some crushed ice and kept fresh with more ice from the hotel ice machine, these milk sub-stitutes can be used for days. (It's a good idea to wrap the mar-garine in a plastic bag so that the melting ice doesn't get all over it.) With a few crushproof bagels packed in my suitcase and a pot of coffee or tea and juice from room service, I have a quick and filling breakfast, more than enough to keep me going until lunchtime. Depending upon your taste, your ingenuity, and the amount of food you want to haul around in your luggage, you can cut your dependence on strange restaurants in half without ever needing a refrigerator or more luggage than a tote bag.

And if you do make a mistake, and your insides rebel . . . In America, there is a book for everything. If you need a bathroom in New York City, you'll undoubtedly want a copy of Lana Toni Gersmon's *Dear John: A Guide to Some of the Best Seats in New York City* (New York: Tribeca Communications, Inc.). Who knows what other helpful items you can find if you search hard enough.

Despite the comfort of knowing such books exist, I never travel without a heaping quantity of lactase pills—some in my luggage and some carried with me, just in case. The reassurance they provide, even if I never need them, makes the whole trip run a lot smoother for me. Taking along lactase is good advice in the United States and absolutely crucial if you travel out of the coun-try. Yes, some manufacturers of lactase pills distribute them over-seas, but you'll find it all too easy to wander into a strange corner of the world where the concept of lactase pills has never been heard of—but milk has.

Into the Unknown with Lactase and Phrase Book

I like to think that I'm not too bad at explaining things in English. Even so, I wish I had a dollar for every time I've been served a dinner roll and butter five minutes after carefully informing a waiter or waitress that I can't have any milk products. Remem-bering times like those makes me shudder at the thought of trav-eling anywhere in the world where good American English is not spoken.

Every year, however, people with worse problems than ours

manage to pull themselves around the world, eating in cheap hotels, strangers' homes, and restaurants that haven't even heard of the fork. I'm not sure how they do it. A smile and a few hand gestures might be enough to get the concept of milk across, but "partially demineralized whey solids" is probably beyond the capacity even of a Marcel Marceau. Try it the next time you play charades and let me know what happens.

Anyway, I'd rather take my chances with a really superior phrase book. What makes for a superior phrase book? I'd say it's one with phrases in several widely used foreign languages covering a variety of realistic situations you're likely to find yourself in. One that describes the differences among various national eating habits. One that gives the names for a long list of milk products. One that gives useful medical information and tips on finding medical aid overseas.

In short, one very like *The Special Diet Foreign Phrase Book*, by Helen Saltz Jacobson (Rodale Press, 1982, $10.95 in paperback). While the book doesn't specifically mention lactose intolerance—or lactose, for that matter—the phrases collected will enable you to order milk-free meals, either off the menu or specially made. Everything in the book is translated four times—into French, German, Italian, and Spanish (with extra phrases for Mexican Spanish where necessary). Four specialty diets are covered: low sodium (low salt); diabetic; low fat and low cholesterol; ulcer, bland, soft, and low residue.

There is also a section on creating your own custom diet, which includes valuable phrases like:

> "Does this dish contain any _____?"
> "Can you prepare this dish without _____?"
> "Are there any dishes on your menu that do not contain ingredients forbidden to me?"
> "A mistake can cause serious illness."

and even

> "Show me on the menu which dishes you can prepare without any of the items on this list."

If you're wondering where to get that handy list, you simply turn to the section in each language listing names of dairy products, including milk, cream, butter, and cheese. If you want to ask specifically for a nondairy creamer, that's in the book, too. This section is slightly different in each language, as each is geared to the individual European country (France, Germany, Italy, and Spain) concerned.

Much, much more is included in the book than I can describe here: mealtimes, tipping, medical aid, emergency telephone numbers, the addresses of the U.S. embassies in each country. There's even a quick guide to pronunciation to help make yourself understood when trying out phrases like *Y a-t-il dans ce plat aucun des ingredients de cette liste*? Not that anything short of a larynx transplant will help you with French vowels. If you're too shy to brazen out a fractured French, just point to the proper phrase. There's even a section for possible replies that the waiter or waitress can point back to. And dollars to deutsch marks, you'll still get a dinner roll and butter delivered to you less than five minutes later.

The Special Diet Foreign Phrase Book does not appear in the 1985 edition of *Books in Print*, so unless a new edition is put out, which I hope happens, you will have to search for it in libraries or used-book stores. It should be well worth the effort.

Attending Carnival Week in Sunny Las Los

French, German, Italian, and Spanish will take you a long way, but what if you get an irresistible urge to vacation in beautiful downtown Zagreb, the second largest city in Yugoslavia? Pointing to *C'e aggiunta di panna* ("Has cream been added?" in Italian) won't do you much good if the maitre d' reads only Serbo-Croatian. When the need arises to say *Ima li ovde neki dobar, jeftin restoran*? ("Can you recommend a good, cheap restaurant?") in Serbo-Croatian or thirteen other languages, the place to turn is Berlitz's *European Menu Reader* (Editions Berlitz, distributed by Macmillan, 1982, $4.95 in paperback), kept in print along with all the dozens of other Berlitz phrase books.

Much more limited in scope than *The Special Diet Foreign Phrase Book*, the *Menu Reader* provides a quick and dirty method of sounding out strange dishes over most of Europe. A guide to pronunciation and a selection of phrases to help you order from a menu are given for Danish, Dutch, Finnish, French, German, Greek, Italian, Norwegian, Polish, Portuguese, Russian, Serbo-Croatian, Spanish, and Swedish. Each section also lists dozens of foods and dishes native to that cuisine, along with descriptions of the contents of those dishes. For example, in Portugal, you would know that *chispalhada*, pig's feet stewed with navy beans, cabbage, bacon, and blood sausage, is probably safe, while *fatias dourades*, slices of bread dipped in milk and egg yolk, fried and sprinkled with sugar, definitely is not.

The *European Menu Master* lists American and British dishes for those two countries separated by a common language. In Britain, baked Alaska is referred to as Norwegian omelet. I don't have a clue as to what it's called in Norway.

LACTOSE AROUND THE WORLD

I do happen to know what lactose is in Norwegian, if the occasion should ever come up: *melkesukker*, which is a literal translation of lactose's other identity, milk sugar. *Lactose* is actually a fairly easy word to translate in most languages. *Lactose* itself is a scientific word, so it stays remarkably constant across language boundaries. Even if it didn't, *milk* and *sugar* are words so common as to be found in almost any dictionary.

Just for fun, here's *lactose* and/or *milk sugar* in more languages than you'll ever need to know.

Afrikaans	*laktose, melksuiker*
French	*lactose, sucre (m) de lait*
German	*laktose, Milchzucker*
Greek	*λῆκτῶς, γαλακτοζάκχαρον*
Italian	*lattosio, zucchero di latte*
Lithuanian	*piencukris*
Norwegian	*melkesukker*
Polish	*laktoza, cukier mlekowy*
Portuguese	*lactose*
Russian	**лактóза, молóчный сáхар**

Serbo-Croatian	*laktoza, mliječni šećer*
Slovene	*laktoza, mlečni sladkor*
Spanish	*azúcar de leche*
Swedish	*mjölksocker*
Tibetan	ཨོ་མའི་ཀ་ར། ཇ་(ཡི་གཟུགས་སོགས་སྐུ)
Ukranian	молочний цукор

OLDIES BUT GOODIES

A number of other menu-translating books exist, all unfortunately out of print. They undoubtedly can still be found in libraries and used-book stores, and language doesn't change that fast anyway. *Eating in Eight Languages* (Stein and Day, 1968, in paperback) by Wilma George is sort of a stripped-down *European Menu Master*. Its eight languages are English, French, Italian, German, Spanish, Portuguese, Greek, and Serbo-Croatian. It shares the *Menu Master*'s disadvantage that the words and phrases are alphabetized in the foreign language. One nice feature is a word-finder in the back of the book in all eight languages, making it easy to find the translations for *milk*, *butter*, and *cheese*.

A very similar book is *Menu Translator*, by Eleanor B. Pierce (Pan American Airways, 1968, in hardback). This book concentrates on countries, listing menu phrases and basic information on the cuisines of Austria, Belgium, Britain, Denmark, Finland, France, Germany, Italy, The Netherlands, Norway, Portugal, Spain, Sweden, and Switzerland.

James Beard's *How to Eat (and Drink) Your Way Through a French (and Italian) Menu* (Atheneum, 1971, in hardback) is staggeringly complete. For nearly two hundred pages, Beard lists virtually every dish you might find in French or Italian cuisine and describes it lovingly. Only one thing is wrong with this book: Who in the world has enough chutzpah to pull it out in an expensive French restaurant?

These are just the books I was able to find with little effort. Many more exist, some even more specialized than Beard's. One is probably right for you.

DR. LIVINGSTONE DOESN'T MAKE HOUSE CALLS

Say you brought along the wrong phrase book and ate something you shouldn't have while in Luxembourg. What then? The book I would turn to first is *Traveling Healthy: A Complete Guide to Medical Services in 23 Countries*, by Sheilah M. Hillman and Robert A. Hillman (Penguin, 1980, in paperback). The authors talk about the availability of doctors, hospitals, and health care in almost every country in Europe plus Israel and Mexico. The information is so complete that they even cite phone numbers and special health services in specific hospitals. Unfortunately the specifics are based on trips the Hillmans took in 1978 and 1979, so much of what they say may well be totally out of date. As a general introduction to health emergencies in foreign countries, however, it has a lot to offer. It, too, is out of print, so some searching will be necessary to find it.

CHAPTER TWELVE

COOKING WITHOUT MILK

To succeed in cooking without milk, you need to know two basics: how to substitute for milk and how to substitute for butter. Once you know these—and these secrets along with several others were revealed in Chapter 6—the majority of all the recipes that were in your everyday diet are yours again. Another large category—recipes with cheese—can be regained if you find that you can tolerate low-lactose ripened cheese, such as Cheddar.

CREAM SAUCE SUBSTITUTES

BASIC SAUCES

Hundreds of dishes you can't eat at a restaurant are available to you at home, including soufflés, casseroles, soups, mousses, and croquettes, once you learn two variations on a crucial basic recipe.

This starter recipe comes in two guises: a "white" sauce and a broth-based variation, known as velouté sauce. These sauces have endless uses:

- Add other ingredients to flavor them and they can be poured over foods as sauces.
- They can be the foundation for casseroles or a seafood mousse.

- Thicken them, and they become binders for making soufflés and croquettes.
- With liquids and cooked vegetables added, they become soups.

A term you'll see in many cream sauce recipes is *roux*. Normally a roux is a mixture of melted butter and flour, cooked and used as a thickener to form the base of the sauce. I'll always substitute a milk-free margarine (not a diet margarine) for the butter.

One hint: always read the entire recipe through before starting. You may find you have to do two or more steps simultaneously, or pull out extra pans or ingredients when you least suspect needing them. A secret of good cooking is to never be surprised at what is coming up next.

Basic White Sauce

    2 tablespoons margarine

    2 tablespoons all-purpose flour

    Dash each salt and pepper

    ½ cup (4 ounces) Coffee Rich*

    ½ cup water

In a small saucepan, melt margarine over low heat. Remove from heat and stir in flour, salt, and pepper until smooth. Slowly stir in Coffee Rich and water. Cook over low heat, stirring constantly, until mixture just comes to a boil. (This will take much longer than you think, and you may want to increase the heat just a little to speed things up.)

Makes 1 cup of sauce.

*All recipes using Coffee Rich are provided by Rich Products Corporation and are used with permission.

Basic Velouté Sauce

    2 tablespoons margarine

    2 tablespoons all-purpose flour

    Dash each salt and pepper

    1 cup chicken broth or stock

In a small saucepan, melt margarine over low heat. Stir flour, salt, and pepper into margarine until smooth and bubbly. Slowly stir in chicken broth. (If you use bouillon from a cube or powder instead of canned or homemade chicken broth, do not add additional salt.) Increase heat and bring to a boil. Boil for 1 minute.
Makes 1 cup of sauce.

For a thicker sauce or a soufflé base, double the ratio of margarine and flour to liquid used in either recipe.

It's difficult, though not impossible, to ruin either sauce. The most common errors are using too high a heat or leaving the sauce unattended on the stove, both of which can cause the sauce to burn. I find I can turn the heat up to medium and stir only occasionally (especially if I'm preparing another part of the meal) without destroying the sauce. You've got to catch it as it starts boiling, however.

A few more hints: Cook the roux for a minute or so before adding the liquid; otherwise you may taste raw flour in the final product. You can increase the ratio of flour to margarine, increase or decrease the ratio of roux to liquid, or add flavoring at any step in the process to create interesting variations (some of which are described in the following recipes) or meet the needs of a particular recipe. Too much margarine unbalanced by flour, however, may make the sauce taste greasy.

The two sauces do have some subtle differences between them. Any plain white sauce is quite bland (some cookbooks compare it to library paste), but this very blandness prevents its taste from competing with the flavors of the added ingredients. Velouté sauce has a stronger intrinsic flavor, from its chicken stock. A white sauce made with Coffee Rich or a similar milk substitute can't be boiled for more than a very short time; long boiling will leave a scorched taste. Velouté sauce is lower in calories and saturated fats than the white sauce (unless a low-saturated-fat milk substitute like Poly Rich or Mocha Mix is used) and will also work to enhance the flavor of meat or vegetables because of the stock or broth used as a base. Chicken croquettes, for example, are best based on a velouté sauce, as the chicken stock improves the flavor of the entire croquette.

BASIC SAUCE VARIATIONS

LEMON WHITE SAUCE: add 2 tablespoons lemon juice when adding Coffee Rich and water.

FLORENTINE SAUCE: add 1 tablespoon lemon juice to the white or velouté sauce. Add ⅓ cup thawed and drained frozen chopped spinach. Heat, stirring constantly. Serve hot over poached or broiled flounder or other white fish.

HORSERADISH SAUCE: add 1 tablespoon horseradish and a few drops Tabasco sauce, or 1 tablespoon horseradish and 1 tablespoon mustard to the finished white or velouté sauce and stir well. Use as sauce on meat.

PARSLEY SAUCE: add ¼ cup minced parsley and 2 well-beaten egg yolks to finished white or velouté sauce. Stir well. Use as sauce on vegetables.

NORMANDY SAUCE: substitute 1 cup fish stock for the chicken stock in the velouté sauce. Add 1 tablespoon lemon juice and 2 well-beaten egg yolks. Stir well. Use as sauce on fish.

BÉCHAMEL SAUCE: use ½ cup milk substitute and ½ cup chicken broth as the sauce liquid. Season with salt, pepper, and paprika.

TOMATO SAUCE: substitute tomato juice for chicken stock in velouté sauce. Add nutmeg, oregano, dry mustard, or basil with the salt and pepper. Use on poultry or eggs.

NEWBURG SAUCE: substitute fish stock for the chicken stock in velouté sauce. Just before serving, stir in 2 slightly beaten egg yolks and 2 tablespoons sherry or 1 tablespoon sherry and 1 tablespoon brandy. Use for shellfish and flaked fish.

BROWN SAUCE: cook roux until lightly browned. Substitute beef consomme for chicken stock in velouté sauce. For flavor, try these optional additions: chopped onion (cooked briefly in the margarine of the roux); dry mustard and curry powder; currant jelly and sherry or port. Use brown or onion sauce for beef, curry sauce for veal or poultry, currant sauce for lamb.

Cream Soup Substitutes

Either white or velouté sauce will work fine as the base of a cream soup, but again there are slight variations in the approach, depending upon the type of soup you're making.

Basic "Cream" Soup

   2 tablespoons minced onion

  ¼ cup (½ stick) margarine

  ¼ cup all-purpose flour

   2 cups (16 ounces) Coffee Rich

1½ cups water

   1 tablespoon instant vegetable broth

  ½ teaspoon lemon juice

In a medium saucepan, sauté onion in margarine. Stir frequently. Cook for about 6 minutes, then remove from heat. Stir in flour, Coffee Rich, water, instant vegetable broth, and lemon juice. Return to medium heat and stir constantly until mixture boils and thickens. Reduce heat. Simmer for 1 minute.

Makes 2 servings.

This basic recipe is more the foundation for the thousands of different cream soups that exist in the world than a soup you would want to make and enjoy for its own sake. I'll just list a few variations here to give you an idea of what is possible. The next step is to open your favorite cookbook and experiment for yourself.

"CREAMY" MUSHROOM SOUP: add 1 jar (4½ ounces) drained sliced mushrooms and ¼ cup chopped parsley to soup base. Simmer for 5 minutes.

BROCCOLI SOUP: add ½ cup thawed and drained frozen chopped broccoli. Simmer for 5 minutes.

HEARTY CORN CHOWDER: sauté ½ cup finely sliced celery and ⅓ cup finely chopped green pepper along with onion in basic recipe. Simmer. Add 1 can (12 ounces) whole kernel corn, drained, with remaining ingredients. Reduce heat and simmer for 8 minutes.

Notice that the basic cream soup recipe starts with sautéing vegetables in margarine and then adding flour and the Coffee Rich. You shouldn't pour a completed white sauce on top of sautéed vegetables because the cream sauce already has margarine in it. The result will be greasy unless you planned ahead by reducing the ratio of margarine to flour in the roux.

Starting with sautéed vegetables is not necessary. If you don't, you can easily make some cream soups by just adding a white or velouté sauce to cooked vegetables and their cooking liquid.

Cream of Tomato Soup

    1 can (28 ounces) peeled crushed tomatoes in puree

    1 medium onion, diced

    1 bay leaf

  1½ cups prepared white or velouté sauce

       Salt and pepper to taste

    1 teaspoon sugar

Combine tomatoes, onion, and bay leaf, and simmer for 10 minutes. Remove bay leaf. Force through sieve to remove tomato seeds. Return mixture to saucepan. Add sauce, salt, pepper, and sugar. Heat through, stirring occasionally. Do not let boil. (You may want to adjust the amount of added sauce to taste.)
Makes 3–4 servings.

Variations on this style of soup include cream soups with meat.

CREAM OF CHICKEN SOUP: add ½ cup chopped cooked chicken and ¼ cup chopped celery or mushrooms to 1 cup chicken broth. Simmer for 15 minutes. Add 1 cup velouté sauce, salt, and pepper. Heat through.

Soups are the individualist's art, created to personal taste by endless tinkering and adjusting. In fact, playing with other people's recipes is almost a commandment when it comes to soup making. From these basics, however, you can make cream soups as thick, hearty, or elegant as you wish.

Casseroles

Both white and velouté sauces or the cream soups they produce can be substituted for the cream of mushroom (or celery or other) soups often found in ordinary casserole recipes.

Easy Tuna–Potato Chip Casserole

    3   tablespoons milk-free margarine
    ¼   cup flour
    1   can (10½ ounces) chicken broth
    ⅓   cup water
    1   celery stalk, diced
    1   can (7–8 ounces) mushrooms, stems and pieces
    2   teaspoons chopped parsley
    1   tablespoon lemon juice
    3   cups crushed potato chips
    2   cans (7 ounces each) water-packed tuna

Melt margarine in a small saucepan. Stir in flour. Cook until bubbly. Add chicken broth, water, celery, mushrooms (including liquid), parsley, and lemon juice. Continue cooking, stirring occasionally, until thickened.

Grease a 2-quart casserole dish. Layer 1 cup of potato chips, half the tuna, flaked, and half the sauce mixture. Repeat layers. Top with potato chips. Microwave at high for 15 to 17 minutes or preheat oven and cook at 350 degrees for 35 minutes, until bubbly.

Once you have the basic cream sauce down pat, go back to your cookbooks and look at those recipes you've been avoiding. Chances are that many of them can be adapted for use with one of these cream-sauce substitutes. Occasionally some experimentation will be necessary to get the proportions and flavors correct: since neither the white nor the velouté sauce tastes exactly like a true cream sauce, you will often have to play with the spices, flavorings, or oils to bring out the full flavor of the foods. The sheer number of old-favorite dishes you can once more bring to your table should more than make up for trade-offs in taste.

CREAM FILLING SUBSTITUTES

Let's not forget desserts while we're substituting. Cream puffs, éclairs, filled cakes, and crepes can again wend their calorie-laden way to your taste buds with a basic cream filling substitute that, as with the sauces, can be used straight or as the basis for many other dishes.

Vanilla "Cream"

½ cup sugar

¼ cup cornstarch

1 cup (8 ounces) Coffee Rich

1 cup water

4 egg yolks, slightly beaten

1 teaspoon vanilla

In a medium saucepan, mix sugar and cornstarch. Stir in Coffee Rich and water. Cook over medium heat, stirring constantly, until mixture boils. Remove from heat. Stir half of hot mixture into egg yolks. Mix well. Return egg mixture to saucepan. Cook, stirring constantly, until mixture is thickened and boiling. Remove from heat. Stir in vanilla. Cool to room temperature. Cover and chill until ready to use.

Makes 4 dessert servings.

You can eat the "cream" straight, or layered with fruits as a parfait. Or you can go on and create other desserts with it.

Boston Cream Pie

1¾ cups cake flour

¼ teaspoon salt

2 teaspoons baking powder

⅓ cup milk-free margarine

    1 cup sugar

    2 eggs

    ½ cup (4 ounces) Coffee Rich

    ½ teaspoon vanilla extract

Stir together flour, salt, and baking powder, and set aside.

In a large bowl, cream together margarine and sugar until light and fluffy. Add eggs, one at a time. Beat well after each addition. Add flour mixture alternately with Coffee Rich, and beat until blended. Stir in vanilla.

Pour batter into 2 lightly greased and floured 8-inch round layer cake pans. Bake in preheated 350-degree oven for 25 to 30 minutes, or until lightly browned. Cool cakes in pans for 5 minutes. Remove and cool on wire racks.

When completely cooled, make ½ Vanilla "Cream" recipe and spread between cake layers. Drizzle chocolate glaze over cake top.

Chocolate glaze

    2 tablespoons milk-free margarine

    1 ounce unsweetened chocolate

    1 cup confectioner's sugar

    1 tablespoon boiling water

In a small saucepan, melt margarine and chocolate, stirring constantly. Remove from heat. Stir in sugar and boiling water. Beat until smooth and thickened. Cool slightly before drizzling on cake.

Everything Else

Many, many recipes can quickly be converted to being lactose free by using the milk, butter, and cream cheese substitutes listed in Chapter 6. Others require more thought or ingenuity. Sometimes a sour cream dish can use plain yogurt in place of the sour cream. If the recipe calls for a cheese sauce, either use a low-lactose, aged cheese or try substituting one of the cream sauce variations mentioned in this chapter. Use your imagination. When all else fails, remember, there is a substitute for everything, even cookbooks.

MILK-FREE COOKBOOKS

Very, very few true milk-free cookbooks for the lactose intolerant exist. If you happen, while wandering through a bookstore or library, to spot a cookbook whose title includes the word *milk free*, chances are that it will be one aimed at people with milk allergies rather than lactose intolerance. Allergies have been a medical issue for years, while understanding of lactose intolerance as a problem is only beginning.

For the most part, you needn't care whom the book is aimed at. Either way, milk free is milk free. In the lists that follow, I've ignored whether the cookbook was written for someone with lactose intolerance or milk allergy. Instead, I've put the cookbooks solely about milk in one group and the ones that mention milk among other food allergies in a second.

Milk-free cookbooks of any sort are tough to find. Some— the few that are in print—either will be at or can be ordered through a good bookstore. For the rest, you'll have to use your ingenuity and go hunting in libraries, used-book stores, or even garage sales. You may find some not listed here: allergy cookbooks come and go very rapidly.

These cookbooks are listed simply as a convenience to you. I'm not recommending any one over the others because I simply don't use them very much. Instead, I rely upon the milk-free substitutes and recipes I talk about in this book to make both the foods I ate before I knew I had lactose intolerance and any new recipes I feel like trying, using cookbooks, friends, magazines, newspapers, and any other sources I can find. Sure, I've eliminated some of the meals I used to eat, but I did that because my tastes have changed and become healthier, not because I can't have milk products.

I have nothing against milk-free cookbooks, and I admit that they can be very handy, especially to people just learning how to cope with a milk-free diet. Having somebody else do the thinking and worrying—figuring out substitutes and equivalents, fussing over the proper proportions, knowing which spices to add or how long things should be cooked—makes the transition period from one style of diet to another far, far easier. In the long run, however, you're better off having access to the thousands and thousands of cookbooks on the market rather than restricting yourself to the handful listed here. Besides, just because they're milk free doesn't necessarily mean that they're good. One of the books (whose title will never escape my lips) contains the worst brownie recipe in the entire world.

If you aren't already familiar with cookbooks in general, you should become so. People with dietary problems often settle for boring, repetitive cookery because they know those meals are safe and they fear the consequences of experimenting, or because they must avoid so many prepared commercial foods. Browsing through cookbooks provides great opportunities for making food more exciting. Almost any cookbook will provide at least a few recipes you'll like, and not knowing how to cook is no excuse for not trying them.

Cookbooks are a thousand times easier to read and follow than computer manuals, and look how many computers there are in our society, many of them operated by people terrified of doing their own cooking. *Cookbook* is a word sometimes used to put down unimaginative, follow-the-numbers, step-by-step approaches to problems. I say great, that's exactly what someone like myself—who can follow instructions but is not very innovative in a kitchen—wants. Place a cookbook in my hands and I'll tackle anything. Leave me to my own devices and I'll come up with a sandwich every time.

Treat these milk-free cookbooks the same way. Every one of them will have something you're bound to go for. A few moments spent flipping through pages will tell you if the author's tastes agree with yours. You don't even have to worry about figuring out a substitute for the milk; it's all been done for you.

Do whatever you need to do to prove to yourself that a lactose-free diet doesn't have to be limiting. Just a few words of warning: You can still get fat eating too many delicious milk-free desserts.

In the following listing, I've added addresses where I could find them, so that you'll be able to write directly to the company if you can't find a bookstore willing to do the ordering for you. No prices are listed because they're too subject to change. Virtually all the books are moderately priced trade paperbacks. The Mead Johnson and Isomil books are actually small pamphlets and are available free from the companies.

Totally Milk-free Cookbooks

ALMOST BUTTER: ALTERNATIVE BUTTER RECIPE BOOK and *ALMOST MILK: MILK FROM NON ANIMAL SOURCES*, by the Alpha Pyramis Research Division Staff (Alpha Pyramis Publishing Co.: send orders to Prosperity and Profits Unlimited, Box 510213, Houston, TX 77257)

COOKING WITH ISOMIL (Ross Laboratories, 625 Cleveland Ave., Columbus, OH 43216)

LIVING . . . WITHOUT MILK, by Jacqueline Hostage, 1981 (Betterway Publications, General Delivery, White Hall, VA 22987)

MEALS WITHOUT MILK, 1981 (Mead Johnson & Company, Department 42, Evansville, IN 47721)

MILK-FREE DIET COOKBOOK, by Jane Zukin, 1981 (Sterling Pub. Co., 2 Park Avenue S., New York, NY 10016)

THE NO MILK COOKBOOK, by Barbara Newby Borgwardt, 1982 (Parkway Publications, Box 19845, West Allis, WI 53219)

Cookbooks Including Milk-free Recipes with Other Food Allergy Recipes

THE ALLERGIC GOURMET, by June Roth, 1983 (Contemporary Books, 180 N. Michigan Avenue, Chicago, IL 60601)

THE ALLERGY BAKER: A COLLECTION OF WHEAT-FREE, MILK-FREE, EGG-FREE, CORN-FREE, AND SOY-FREE RECIPES, by Carol Rudoff, 1980. Also, *THE ALLERGY GOURMET: A COLLECTION OF WHEAT-FREE, MILK-FREE, EGG-FREE, CORN-FREE, AND SOY-FREE RECIPES,* by Carol Rudoff, 1983. (Both from Prologue Publications, Box 640, Menlo Park, CA 94026)

THE ALLERGY COOKBOOK: TASTY NUTRITIOUS COOKING WITHOUT WHEAT, CORN, MILK & EGGS, by Ruth Shattuck, 1984 (NAL, New York)

THE ALLERGY COOKBOOK & FOOD BUYING GUIDE, by Pamela P. Nonken and S. Roger Hirsch, 1982 (Warner Books, NY)

THE EGG FREE, MILK FREE, WHEAT FREE COOKBOOK, by Becky Hamrick, 1981 (Cygnus Press, Midland, TX)

GOOD FOOD, MILK FREE, GRAIN FREE, by Hilda Cherry Hills, 1980 (Keats Publishing, 27 Pine Street, New Canaan, CT, 06480)

THE MILK-FREE AND MILK-FREE EGG-FREE COOKBOOK, by Isobel S. Sainsbury, 1979 (Arco, Division of Prentice-Hall, 215 Park Avenue S., New York, NY 10003)

WHEAT-FREE, MILK-FREE, EGG-FREE COOKING, by Rita Greer 1984, (Thorsons Publishing, New York, Distributed by Inner Traditions International, 377 Park Avenue S., New York, NY 10016)

CHAPTER THIRTEEN

ASSERTING YOUR RIGHTS

If you do decide to give up lactose entirely, you'll find that the world is not designed for the lactose intolerant. The information you so desperately need to make the proper choices is often simply not available, from anyone. Worse, you can get fooled by foods and medicines that you thought were safe but prove to contain lactose.

Demanding more information is your right as a consumer. This final chapter should give you a few ideas on how to stand up for those rights and make a lactose-free life easier and more pleasurable.

ASK, ASK, AND ASK AGAIN

Most packaged foods and drugs now come with ingredients lists printed on their labels. Without these lists, shopping for commercial foods and common medications would be almost impossible; give thanks to all those who fought to get ingredients labeling as widely used as it is. Unfortunately, the lists are still not perfect. For example, how can you know if the margarine or semisweet chocolate listed on some food packages contains any milk unless the label is specific enough to tell you so? The only way to find out is to write to that company and ask.

Most companies are very willing to supply lists of the products they make without lactose. Even the ones that aren't are usually willing to answer questions about individual foods they make. Many will reward you for being interested in their products by sending along coupons or recipe booklets. Just by the act of writing, you'll let them know of your interest in lactose-free products, which will weigh heavily with that company the next time it decides which other products to market.

Some of the larger companies have toll-free 800 numbers that will connect you directly with their consumer information departments. These numbers may be printed on the labels of the products they sell, or you can call 1-800-555-1212 free and ask if a particular company has a toll-free number.

Even when the companies have lists prepared in anticipation of your question, you can't always be sure that the lists are correct. Old products are removed from the market, new ones get added, and the recipes for any products, even old favorites, are subject to change without notice. The lactose-free product lists don't always keep up with these changes. Occasionally, too, products that have and have always had milk products get included on these lists. If you find that a company's lists are incorrect, you should contact the company's consumer affairs department and let them know. The lists are a great service and may alert you to many products you may not have considered before, but they are no substitute for checking the ingredients lists on any packaged food before you buy it.

Drugs almost always come packaged, but foods may not. Stores are not obligated to label unpackaged foods. The bakery, delicatessen, or bulk food section of a supermarket is probably filled with foods that are lactose-free without any labels to let you know that this is the case. Start with the store managers and see if they have the proper information. If not, many supermarket chains have consumer information telephone numbers of their own. When you ask for information, remind the person you talk to that accurate, adequate labeling would be a big help to those of us who are lactose intolerant. Emphasize that labeling would make a difference when you decide where to shop.

SUPPORT LACTOSE-FREE PRODUCTS

Large companies care about their customers' interests, but they care even more about their bottom lines. Buying lactose-free products is a good start. (You would, if you're trying to keep to a strict milk-free diet, buy those products anyway.) A better step is to buy those products that advertise themselves as having no lactose, especially if a similar product on the market is also lactose free but doesn't say so. The best action of all is to let the manufacturer know that the reason you are buying its products is precisely that they are lactose free, and that you would buy others of its products if they were lactose free as well.

Manufacturers rarely get as much feedback from their customers as they would like, so making a point about why you are buying that company's products and not its competitors' will have real impact. If enough people did so, the manufacturer would have to think very carefully when changing the ingredients in its products or creating something new. Don't expect a cheese sauce to disappear if that's the main selling point of a food, but a large consumer response would help accelerate the trend toward increasing the number of products aimed at the lactose-intolerant market.

One other piece of labeling that you should request of manufacturers is a *no-lactose* or *lactose-free* label placed somewhere on the package. You can suggest that you would make a point of buying those products with such labels, since they would save you the chore of having to read ingredients lists over and over to make sure that some milk product wasn't snuck in when you weren't looking. A consistent, industry-wide symbol would be nice, but working on manufacturers one by one at first is likely to get more results. Remember, don't be afraid to let manufacturers know how many of you are out there. Once they realize that the lactose intolerant are a market that is large enough to be worth catering to, we'll see more and more concessions made toward our existence.

What I say about manufacturers is true of restaurants as well. They are as concerned as any other business about satisfying their customers. Patronize those restaurants that have a great many lactose-free meals on the menu or those that will cheerfully make foods specially for you. A restaurant near me has foods checked on its menu that the chef will cook without butter on request. This service is aimed at calorie counters, but it works just as well for the lactose intolerant. It's a simple, convenient idea that could easily be copied by many more restaurants if they realized that many of their customers desired it.

COMPLAIN

For the lactose intolerant, the most confusing label on packaged foods is *nondairy*. The presence of this label is required by several dairy states when a food contains sodium caseinate but no other milk product. The U.S. Food and Drug Administration (FDA) accepts this labeling because, as FDA Associate Commissioner for Regulatory Affairs Joesph P. Hile has said, "we believe it is important that products which contain sodium caseinate but no other ingredients commonly found in or derived from milk be marketed for what they are and that their labeling should in no way suggest or imply that they are the normal products made from milk or cream."

The presence of pure sodium caseinate (a protein) in foods is not a problem to the lactose intolerant, but manufacturers don't always stop at sodium caseinate in foods listed as nondairy. Some also add true milk products such as whey. The FDA does not allow this and will contact the firm responsible and ask it to correct the labeling if someone tells the FDA about the violation.

To get the FDA to act on such a complaint, remove the label from a product you believe to be mislabeled and send it to the Consumer Affairs Officer at your regional FDA office (whose address should be available in the section under U.S. Government Agencies in your phone book). Doing so will give the FDA the proof they need to confront the guilty party.

Any other complaints about packaged foods and drugs should be addressed to the FDA as well. In addition, the organization is a great repository of information that will answer many of the questions you may have about foods and drugs. Make it work for you.

YOUR ELECTED OFFICIALS WORK FOR YOU

Maybe the FDA has no authority over state laws, but the governor and legislature in your state certainly do. If you live in a state with "nondairy" laws, then you should write to your representatives in the legislature and strongly suggest to them that such laws are outmoded.

Perhaps the FDA should be urged to eliminate some of the loopholes in their labeling regulations. That's a national concern, one you should contact your senator or representative in Congress to express. In fact, any ideas you have for better consumer protection should be passed along to the proper elected officials. Labeling is required on packaged foods, but why shouldn't fast-food chains, with their standardized menus, also have to post ingredients for their products? Why shouldn't all pharmaceutical manufacturers be required to list inactive ingredients on their labels rather than trusting to the voluntary labeling being practiced by some, but not all, firms? Why shouldn't there be a single standard for measuring the activity of lactase enzyme, so that the strengths of the various lactase pills can be directly compared?

Once again, the presence of a large group of lactose-intolerant individuals, and the problems we face, is almost unknown in this country. If elected officials aren't made aware of our numbers, we'll never see any legislation to help cure our frustrations. The answer to any consumer problem is to make yourself heard, let your concerns be aired, and be sure that everyone you contact understands that you represent large numbers of others with the same concerns.

SOURCES OF INFORMATION ON LACTOSE INTOLERANCE

Lactose Digestion: Clinical and Nutritional Implications, edited by David M. Paige and Theodore M. Bayless (Baltimore: The Johns Hopkins University Press, 1981).

Milk Intolerances and Rejection, edited by J. Delmont (Basel: S. Karger, 1983).

These are the only other books on the subject of lactose intolerance I am aware of. Both are collections of articles on the subject by doctors, scientists, and other health care professionals, and are aimed at a similar audience. They make for extremely difficult reading. If I had to choose one, it would be the Paige and Bayless book, because its articles give a somewhat better overview of the field. The books are likely to be found only in the libraries of large medical schools.

In the Matter of California Milk Producers Advisory Board, Et Al., Federal Trade Commission Decisions, 94 F.T.C. 429 (1979)

The FTC versus the group behind the slogan Every Body Needs Milk. What about the lactose intolerant? asked the FTC, and brought the country's top medical experts on lactose intolerance in front of Administrative Law Judge Daniel H. Hanscom to argue the facts. Judge Hanscom's decision, which summarizes the testimony at great length, is a fascinating and readable document filled with information on America's nutritional habits, faulty scientific research, mass media marketing, and even lactose intolerance. Although the judge finds against the FTC in the end, making light of our problems, his scrupulous presentation of the hearing is worth the reading.

Allergies to Milk, by Sami L. Bahna and Douglas C. Heiner (New York: Grune & Stratton, 1980).

In this, the only book entirely devoted to milk-produced allergies, lactose intolerance is mentioned only as an aside. Not only that, but *Allergies to Milk* is as extremely technical as the Paige and Bayless and Delmont volumes. Since milk allergy is primarily a problem of young children, however, this book has a very different focus from the others, and its section on milk substitutes and milk-free recipes is valuable in its own right.

Newer Knowledge of Milk and other Fluid Dairy Products, National Dairy Council (Rosemont, IL 60018, 1978).

Milk and Milk Products in Human Nutrition, second edition revised, by S. K. Kon (FAO Nutritional Studies No. 27, Food and Agricultural Organization of the United Nations, Rome, 1972).

Both of these books do a good job of explaining the role and value of milk in nutrition, making convincing arguments for why you should continue to drink milk if you can still do so. The National Dairy Council booklet is by far the more readable.

A listing of milk-free cookbooks can be found at the end of Chapter 12.

NUTRITIVE VALUES OF FOODS

Food values tables are like coffee table books, filled with fascinatingly bizarre information hardly anyone ever bothers to read. For the lactose intolerant, however, such tables are very useful. They can quickly clue you in on foods that are high in the nutrients missing from your diet if you don't eat any milk products.

With this particular table of the more common nutrients, all you need do is follow a column for a particular nutrient, say, riboflavin, from page to page, looking for the foods with the highest numbers (unless, that is, they turn out to be or contain milk products). Wheat flour turns out to be high in riboflavin, and so do green vegetables like broccoli, asparagus, and spinach. You do, however, have to watch that you don't compare apples with oranges, so to speak. A whole apple pie is high in riboflavin, but eating a whole apple pie at a sitting just for its riboflavin content is silly. That's the other advantage of this food values table. You can see at a glance that an apple pie also contains 2,240 calories and five times as much fat as protein, rather reducing its healthfulness.

By balancing the useful nutrients against those you want to reduce in your diet (like calories and fats, especially saturated fats), you'll be able to see how healthy your present diet is and whether you need to add any new foods to your diet to maintain a better nutrition balance. To do a quick check for the foods you currently eat, there is an alphabetical index of the foods listed at the end of the table on page 278.

This table is adapted from *Nutritive Value of Foods*, by Catherine F. Adams and Martha Richardson, prepared by the Science and Education Administration, United States Department of Agriculture, revised edition, April 1981.

NUTRITIVE VALUES OF THE EDIBLE PART OF FOODS

(Dashes (—) denote lack of reliable data for a constituent believed to be present in measurable amount)

Item No. (A)	Foods, approximate measures, units, and weight (edible part unless footnotes indicate otherwise) (B)		Water (C)	Food energy (D)	Protein (E)
			Grams	Percent	Calories	Grams
	DAIRY PRODUCTS (CHEESE, CREAM, IMITATION CREAM, MILK; RELATED PRODUCTS)					
	Butter. See Fats, oils; related products, items 103-108.					
	Cheese:					
	Natural:					
1	Blue------------------------	1 oz------------------------	28	42	100	6
2	Camembert (3 wedges per 4-oz container).	1 wedge---------------------	38	52	115	8
	Cheddar:					
3	Cut pieces-----------------	1 oz------------------------	28	37	115	7
4		1 cu in--------------------	17.2	37	70	4
5	Shredded-------------------	1 cup----------------------	113	37	455	28
	Cottage (curd not pressed down):					
	Creamed (cottage cheese, 4% fat):					
6	Large curd--------------	1 cup----------------------	225	79	235	28
7	Small curd--------------	1 cup----------------------	210	79	220	26
8	Low fat (2%)------------	1 cup----------------------	226	79	205	31
9	Low fat (1%)------------	1 cup----------------------	226	82	165	28
10	Uncreamed (cottage cheese dry curd, less than 1/2% fat).	1 cup----------------------	145	80	125	25
11	Cream-----------------------	1 oz------------------------	28	54	100	2
	Mozzarella, made with—					
12	Whole milk-----------------	1 oz------------------------	28	48	90	6
13	Part skim milk-------------	1 oz------------------------	28	49	80	8
	Parmesan, grated:					
14	Cup, not pressed down------	1 cup----------------------	100	18	455	42
15	Tablespoon----------------	1 tbsp---------------------	5	18	25	2
16	Ounce---------------------	1 oz------------------------	28	18	130	12
17	Provolone-------------------	1 oz------------------------	28	41	100	7
	Ricotta, made with—					
18	Whole milk-----------------	1 cup----------------------	246	72	430	28
19	Part skim milk-------------	1 cup----------------------	246	74	340	28
20	Romano---------------------	1 oz------------------------	28	31	110	9
21	Swiss----------------------	1 oz------------------------	28	37	105	8
	Pasteurized process cheese:					
22	American-------------------	1 oz------------------------	28	39	105	6
23	Swiss----------------------	1 oz------------------------	28	42	95	7
24	Pasteurized process cheese food, American.	1 oz------------------------	28	43	95	6
25	Pasteurized process cheese spread, American.	1 oz------------------------	28	48	80	5
	Cream, sweet:					
26	Half-and-half (cream and milk)-	1 cup----------------------	242	81	315	7
27		1 tbsp---------------------	15	81	20	Trace
28	Light, coffee, or table-------	1 cup----------------------	240	74	470	6
29		1 tbsp---------------------	15	74	30	Trace
	Whipping, unwhipped (volume about double when whipped):					
30	Light-----------------------	1 cup----------------------	239	64	700	5
31		1 tbsp---------------------	15	64	45	Trace
32	Heavy-----------------------	1 cup----------------------	238	58	820	5
33		1 tbsp---------------------	15	58	80	Trace
34	Whipped topping, (pressurized)-	1 cup----------------------	60	61	155	2
35		1 tbsp---------------------	3	61	10	Trace
36	Cream, sour----------------------	1 cup----------------------	230	71	495	7
37		1 tbsp---------------------	12	71	25	Trace
	Cream products, imitation (made with vegetable fat):					
	Sweet:					
	Creamers:					
38	Liquid (frozen)-----------	1 cup----------------------	245	77	335	2
39		1 tbsp---------------------	15	77	20	Trace

[1]Vitamin A value is largely from beta-carotene used for coloring. Riboflavin value for items 40-41 apply to products with added riboflavin.

Fat	Saturated (total)	Oleic	Linoleic	Carbohydrate	Calcium	Phosphorus	Iron	Potassium	Vitamin A value	Thiamin	Riboflavin	Niacin	Ascorbic acid
(F)	(G)	(H)	(I)	(J)	(K)	(L)	(M)	(N)	(O)	(P)	(Q)	(R)	(S)
Grams	Grams	Grams	Grams	Grams	Milligrams	Milligrams	Milligrams	Milligrams	International units	Milligrams	Milligrams	Milligrams	Milligrams
8	5.3	1.9	0.2	1	150	110	0.1	73	200	0.01	0.11	0.3	0
9	5.8	2.2	.2	Trace	147	132	.1	71	350	.01	.19	.2	0
9	6.1	2.1	.2	Trace	204	145	.2	28	300	.01	.11	Trace	0
6	3.7	1.3	.1	Trace	124	88	.1	17	180	Trace	.06	Trace	0
37	24.2	8.5	.7	1	815	579	.8	111	1,200	.03	.42	.1	0
10	6.4	2.4	.2	6	135	297	.3	190	370	.05	.37	.3	Trace
9	6.0	2.2	.2	6	126	277	.3	177	340	.04	.34	.3	Trace
4	2.8	1.0	.1	8	155	340	.4	217	160	.05	.42	.3	Trace
2	1.5	.5	.1	6	138	302	.3	193	80	.05	.37	.3	Trace
1	.4	.1	Trace	3	46	151	.3	47	40	.04	.21	.2	0
10	6.2	2.4	.2	1	23	30	.3	34	400	Trace	.06	Trace	0
7	4.4	1.7	.2	1	163	117	.1	21	260	Trace	.08	Trace	0
5	3.1	1.2	.1	1	207	149	.1	27	180	.01	.10	Trace	0
30	19.1	7.7	.3	4	1,376	807	1.0	107	700	.05	.39	.3	0
2	1.0	.4	Trace	Trace	69	40	Trace	5	40	Trace	.02	Trace	0
9	5.4	2.2	.1	1	390	229	.3	30	200	.01	.11	.1	0
8	4.8	1.7	.1	1	214	141	.1	39	230	.01	.09	Trace	0
32	20.4	7.1	.7	7	509	389	.9	257	1,210	.03	.48	.3	0
19	12.1	4.7	.5	13	669	449	1.1	308	1,060	.05	.46	.2	0
8	—	—	—	1	302	215	—	—	160	—	.11	Trace	0
8	5.0	1.7	.2	1	272	171	Trace	31	240	.01	.10	Trace	0
9	5.6	2.1	.2	Trace	174	211	.1	46	340	.01	.10	Trace	0
7	4.5	1.7	.1	1	219	216	.2	61	230	Trace	.08	Trace	0
7	4.4	1.7	.1	2	163	130	.2	79	260	.01	.13	Trace	0
6	3.8	1.5	.1	2	159	202	.1	69	220	.01	.12	Trace	0
28	17.3	7.0	.6	10	254	230	.2	314	260	.08	.36	.2	2
2	1.1	.4	Trace	1	16	14	Trace	19	20	.01	.02	Trace	Trace
46	28.8	11.7	1.0	9	231	192	.1	292	1,730	.08	.36	.1	2
3	1.8	.7	.1	1	14	12	Trace	18	110	Trace	.02	Trace	Trace
74	46.2	18.3	1.5	7	166	146	0.1	231	2.690	0.06	0.30	0.1	1
5	2.9	1.1	.1	Trace	10	9	Trace	15	170	Trace	.02	Trace	Trace
88	54.8	22.2	2.0	7	154	149	.1	179	3,500	.05	.26	.1	1
6	3.5	1.4	.1	Trace	10	9	Trace	11	220	Trace	.02	Trace	Trace
13	8.3	3.4	.3	7	61	54	Trace	88	550	.02	.04	Trace	0
1	.4	.2	Trace	Trace	3	3	Trace	4	30	Trace	Trace	Trace	0
48	30.0	12.1	1.1	10	268	195	.1	331	1,820	.08	.34	.2	2
3	1.6	.6	.1	1	14	10	Trace	17	90	Trace	.02	Trace	Trace
24	22.8	.3	Trace	28	23	157	.1	467	[1]220	0	0	0	0
1	1.4	Trace	0	2	1	10	Trace	29	[1]10	0	0	0	0

NUTRITIVE VALUES OF THE EDIBLE PART OF FOODS · Continued

(Dashes (—) denote lack of reliable data for a constituent believed to be present in measurable amount)

Item No. (A)	Foods, approximate measures, units, and weight (edible part unless footnotes indicate otherwise) (B)		Water (C)	Food energy (D)	Pro- tein (E)
			Grams	Per- cent	Cal- ories	Grams

DAIRY PRODUCTS (CHEESE, CREAM, IMITATION CREAM, MILK; RELATED PRODUCTS)—Con.

	Cream products, imitation (made with vegetable fat)—Continued Sweet—Continued Creamers—Continued				
40	Powdered-------------------	1 cup----------------------	94	2	515	5
41		1 tsp----------------------	2	2	10	Trace
	Whipped topping:				
42	Frozen---------------------	1 cup----------------------	75	50	240	1
43		1 tbsp---------------------	4	50	15	Trace
44	Powdered, made with whole milk.	1 cup----------------------	80	67	150	3
45		1 tbsp---------------------	4	67	10	Trace
46	Pressurized----------------	1 cup----------------------	70	60	185	1
47		1 tbsp---------------------	4	60	10	Trace
48	Sour dressing (imitation sour cream) made with nonfat dry milk.	1 cup----------------------	235	75	415	8
49		1 tbsp---------------------	12	75	20	Trace
	Ice cream. See Milk desserts, frozen (items 75-80).				
	Ice milk. See Milk desserts, frozen (items 81-83).				
	Milk: Fluid:				
50	Whole (3.3% fat)-------------	1 cup----------------------	244	88	150	8
	Lowfat (2%):				
51	No milk solids added-------	1 cup----------------------	244	89	120	8
	Milk solids added:				
52	Label claim less than 10 g of protein per cup.	1 cup----------------------	245	89	125	9
53	Label claim 10 or more grams of protein per cup (protein fortified).	1 cup----------------------	246	88	135	10
	Lowfat (1%):				
54	No milk solids added------	1 cup----------------------	244	90	100	8
	Milk solids added:				
55	Label claim less than 10 g of protein per cup.	1 cup----------------------	245	90	105	9
56	Label claim 10 or more grams of protein per cup (protein forti- fied).	1 cup----------------------	246	89	120	10
	Nonfat (skim):				
57	No milk solids added------	1 cup----------------------	245	91	85	8
	Milk solids added:				
58	Label claim less than 10 g of protein per cup.	1 cup----------------------	245	90	90	9
59	Label claim 10 or more grams of protein per cup (protein forti- fied).	1 cup----------------------	246	89	100	10
60	Buttermilk------------------	1 cup----------------------	245	90	100	8
	Canned: Evaporated, unsweetened:				
61	Whole milk----------------	1 cup----------------------	252	74	340	17

[1]Vitamin A value is largely from beta-carotene used for coloring. Riboflavin value for items 40-41 apply to products with added riboflavin.
[2]Applies to product without added vitamin A. With added vitamin A, value is 500 International Units (I.U.).
[3]Applies to product without vitamin A added.

Fat	Satu-rated (total)	Unsaturated Oleic	Lino-leic	Carbo-hydrate	Calcium	Phos-phorus	Iron	Potas-sium	Vitamin A value	Thiamin	Ribo-flavin	Niacin	Ascorbic acid
(F)	(G)	(H)	(I)	(J)	(K)	(L)	(M)	(N)	(O)	(P)	(Q)	(R)	(S)
Grams	Grams	Grams	Grams	Grams	Milli-grams	Milli-grams	Milli-grams	Milli-grams	Inter-national units	Milli-grams	Milli-grams	Milli-grams	Milli-grams
33	30.6	.9	Trace	52	21	397	.1	763	[1]190	0	[1].16	0	0
1	.7	Trace	0	1	Trace	8	Trace	16	[1]Trace	0	[1]Trace	0	0
19	16.3	1.0	.2	17	5	6	.1	14	[1]650	0	0	0	0
1	.9	.1	Trace	1	Trace	Trace	Trace	1	[1]30	0	0	0	0
10	8.5	.6	.1	13	72	69	Trace	121	[1]290	.02	.09	Trace	1
Trace	.4	Trace	Trace	1	4	3	Trace	6	[1]10	Trace	Trace	Trace	Trace
16	13.2	1.4	.2	11	4	13	Trace	13	[1]330	0	0	0	0
1	.8	.1	Trace	1	Trace	1	Trace	1	[1]20	0	0	0	0
39	31.2	4.4	1.1	11	266	205	.1	380	[1]20	.09	.38	.2	2
2	1.6	.2	.1	1	14	10	Trace	19	[1]Trace	.01	.02	Trace	Trace
8	5.1	2.1	.2	11	291	228	.1	370	[2]310	.09	.40	.2	2
5	2.9	1.2	.1	12	297	232	.1	377	500	.10	.40	.2	2
5	2.9	1.2	.1	12	313	245	.1	397	500	.10	.42	.2	2
5	3.0	1.2	.1	14	352	276	.1	447	500	.11	.48	.2	3
3	1.6	.7	.1	12	300	235	.1	381	500	.10	.41	.2	2
2	1.5	.6	.1	12	313	245	.1	397	500	.10	.42	.2	2
3	1.8	.7	.1	14	349	273	.1	444	500	.11	.47	.2	3
Trace	.3	.1	Trace	12	302	247	.1	406	500	.09	.34	.2	2
1	0.4	0.1	Trace	12	316	255	0.1	418	500	0.10	0.43	0.2	2
1	.4	.1	Trace	14	352	275	.1	446	500	.11	.48	.2	3
2	1.3	.5	Trace	12	285	219	.1	371	[3]80	.08	.38	.1	2
19	11.6	5.3	0.4	25	657	510	.5	764	[3]610	.12	.80	.5	5

NUTRITIVE VALUES OF THE EDIBLE PART OF FOODS · Continued

(Dashes (—) denote lack of reliable data for a constituent believed to be present in measurable amount)

Item No. (A)	Foods, approximate measures, units, and weight (edible part unless footnotes indicate otherwise) (B)		Water (C)	Food energy (D)	Pro-tein (E)
		Grams	Per-cent	Cal-ories	Grams

DAIRY PRODUCTS (CHEESE, CREAM, IMITATION CREAM, MILK; RELATED PRODUCTS)—Con.

	Milk—Continued				
	Canned—Continued				
	Evaporated, unsweetened—Continued				
62	Skim milk------------------ 1 cup---------------------	255	79	200	19
63	Sweetened, condensed--------- 1 cup---------------------	306	27	980	24
	Dried:				
64	Buttermilk-------------------- 1 cup---------------------	120	3	465	41
	Nonfat instant:				
65	Envelope, net wt., 3.2 oz⁵- 1 envelope---------------	91	4	325	32
66	Cup⁷---------------------- 1 cup---------------------	68	4	245	24
	Milk beverages:				
	Chocolate milk (commercial):				
67	Regular-------------------- 1 cup---------------------	250	82	210	8
68	Lowfat (2%)---------------- 1 cup---------------------	250	84	180	8
69	Lowfat (1%)---------------- 1 cup---------------------	250	85	160	8
70	Eggnog (commercial)----------- 1 cup---------------------	254	74	340	10
	Malted milk, home-prepared with 1 cup of whole milk and 2 to 3 heaping tsp of malted milk powder (about 3/4 oz):				
71	Chocolate-------------------- 1 cup of milk plus 3/4 oz of powder.	265	81	235	9
72	Natural---------------------- 1 cup of milk plus 3/4 oz of powder.	265	81	235	11
	Shakes, thick:⁸				
73	Chocolate, container, net wt., 10.6 oz. 1 container---------------	300	72	355	9
74	Vanilla, container, net wt., 11 oz. 1 container---------------	313	74	350	12
	Milk desserts, frozen:				
	Ice cream:				
	Regular (about 11% fat):				
75	Hardened-------------------- 1/2 gal--------------------	1,064	61	2,155	38
76	1 cup---------------------	133	61	270	5
77	3-fl oz container---------	50	61	100	2
78	Soft serve (frozen custard) 1 cup---------------------	173	60	375	7
79	Rich (about 16% fat), hardened. 1/2 gal--------------------	1,188	59	2,805	33
80	1 cup---------------------	148	59	350	4
	Ice milk:				
81	Hardened (about 4.3% fat)---- 1/2 gal--------------------	1,048	69	1,470	41
82	1 cup---------------------	131	69	185	5
83	Soft serve (about 2.6% fat) 1 cup---------------------	175	70	225	8
84	Sherbet (about 2% fat)------- 1/2 gal--------------------	1,542	66	2,160	17
85	1 cup---------------------	193	66	270	2
	Milk desserts, other:				
86	Custard, baked--------------- 1 cup---------------------	265	77	305	14
	Puddings:				
	From home recipe:				
	Starch base:				
87	Chocolate-------------- 1 cup---------------------	260	66	385	8ˊ
88	Vanilla (blancmange)--- 1 cup---------------------	255	76	285	9
89	Tapioca cream----------- 1 cup---------------------	165	72	220	8
	From mix (chocolate) and milk:				
90	Regular (cooked)--------- 1 cup---------------------	260	70	320	9
91	Instant------------------ 1 cup---------------------	260	69	325	8

³Applies to product without vitamin A added.
⁴Applies to product with added vitamin A. Without added vitamin A, value is 20 International Units (I.U.).
⁵Yields 1 qt of fluid milk when reconstituted according to package directions.
⁶Applies to product with added vitamin A.
⁷Weight applies to product with label claim of 1 1/3 cups equal 3.2 oz.
⁸Applies to products made from thick shake mixes and that do not contain added ice cream.
Products made from milk shake mixes are higher in fat and usually contain added ice cream.

	NUTRIENTS IN INDICATED QUANTITY												
	Fatty Acids												
Fat	Satu-rated (total)	Unsaturated		Carbo-hydrate	Calcium	Phos-phorus	Iron	Potas-sium	Vitamin A value	Thiamin	Ribo-flavin	Niacin	Ascorbic acid
		Oleic	Lino-leic										
(F)	(G)	(H)	(I)	(J)	(K)	(L)	(M)	(N)	(O)	(P)	(Q)	(R)	(S)
Grams	Grams	Grams	Grams	Grams	Milli-grams	Milli-grams	Milli-grams	Milli-grams	Inter-national units	Milli-grams	Milli-grams	Milli-grams	Milli-grams
1	.3	.1	Trace	29	738	497	.7	845	⁴1,000	.11	.79	.4	3
27	16.8	6.7	.7	166	868	775	.6	1,136	³1,000	.28	1.27	.6	8
7	4.3	1.7	.2	59	1,421	1,119	.4	1,910	³260	.47	1.90	1.1	7
1	.4	.1	Trace	47	1,120	896	.3	1,552	⁶2,160	.38	1.59	.8	5
Trace	.3	.1	Trace	35	837	670	.2	1,160	⁶1,610	.28	1.19	.6	4
8	5.3	2.2	.2	26	280	251	.6	417	³300	.09	.41	.3	2
5	3.1	1.3	.1	26	284	254	.6	422	500	.10	.42	.3	2
3	1.5	.7	.1	26	287	257	.6	426	500	.10	.40	.2	2
19	11.3	5.0	.6	34	330	278	.5	420	890	.09	.48	.3	4
9	5.5	—	—	29	304	265	.5	500	330	.14	.43	.7	2
10	6.0	—	—	27	347	307	.3	529	380	.20	.54	1.3	2
8	5.0	2.0	.2	63	396	378	.9	672	260	.14	.67	.4	0
9	5.9	2.4	.2	56	457	361	.3	572	360	.09	.61	.5	0
115	71.3	28.8	2.6	254	1,406	1,075	1.0	2,052	4,340	.42	2.63	1.1	6
14	8.9	3.6	.3	32	176	134	.1	257	540	.05	.33	.1	1
5	3.4	1.4	.1	12	66	51	Trace	96	200	.02	.12	.1	Trace
23	13.5	5.9	.6	38	236	199	.4	338	790	.08	.45	.2	1
190	118.3	47.8	4.3	256	1,213	927	.8	1,771	7,200	.36	2.27	.9	5
24	14.7	6.0	.5	32	151	115	.1	221	900	.04	.28	.1	1
45	28.1	11.3	1.0	232	1,409	1,035	1.5	2,117	1,710	.61	2.78	.9	6
6	3.5	1.4	.1	29	176	129	.1	265	210	.08	.35	.1	1
5	2.9	1.2	0.1	38	274	202	0.3	412	180	0.12	0.54	0.2	1
31	19.0	7.7	.7	469	827	594	2.5	1,585	1,480	.26	.71	1.0	31
4	2.4	1.0	.1	59	103	74	.3	198	190	.03	.09	.1	4
15	6.8	5.4	.7	29	297	310	1.1	387	930	.11	.50	.3	1
12	7.6	3.3	.3	67	250	255	1.3	445	390	.05	.36	.3	1
10	6.2	2.5	.2	41	298	232	Trace	352	410	.08	.41	.3	2
8	4.1	2.5	.5	28	173	180	.7	223	480	.07	.30	.2	2
8	4.3	2.6	.2	59	265	247	.8	354	340	.05	.39	.3	2
7	3.6	2.2	.3	63	374	237	1.3	335	340	.08	.39	.3	2

NUTRITIVE VALUES OF THE EDIBLE PART OF FOODS · Continued

(Dashes (—) denote lack of reliable data for a constituent believed to be present in measurable amount)

Item No. (A)	Foods, approximate measures, units, and weight (edible part unless footnotes indicate otherwise) (B)		Water (C)	Food energy (D)	Protein (E)
		Grams	Per-cent	Cal-ories	Grams

DAIRY PRODUCTS (CHEESE, CREAM, IMITAT`ON CREAM, MILK; RELATED PRODUCTS)—Con.

	Yogurt:				
	With added milk solids:				
	Made with lowfat milk:				
92	Fruit-flavored[9]----------	1 container, net wt., 8 oz	227	75	230	10
93	Plain--------------------	1 container, net wt., 8 oz	227	85	145	12
94	Made with nonfat milk------	1 container, net wt., 8 oz	227	85	125	13
	Without added milk solids:				
95	Made with whole milk-------	1 container, net wt., 8 oz	227	88	140	8

EGGS

	Eggs, large (24 oz per dozen):				
	Raw:				
96	Whole, without shell-------	1 egg---------------------	50	75	80	6
97	White--------------------	1 white-------------------	33	88	15	3
98	Yolk---------------------	1 yolk--------------------	17	49	65	3
	Cooked:				
99	Fried in butter-----------	1 egg---------------------	46	72	85	5
100	Hard-cooked, shell removed_	1 egg---------------------	50	75	80	6
101	Poached------------------	1 egg---------------------	50	74	80	6
102	Scrambled (milk added) in butter. Also omelet.	1 egg---------------------	64	76	95	6

FATS, OILS; RELATED PRODUCTS

	Butter:				
	Regular (1 brick or 4 sticks per lb):				
103	Stick (1/2 cup)-----------	1 stick--------------------	113	16	815	1
104	Tablespoon (about 1/8 stick).	1 tbsp--------------------	14	16	100	Trace
105	Pat (1 in square, 1/3 in high; 90 per lb).	1 pat---------------------	5	16	35	Trace
	Whipped (6 sticks or two 8-oz containers per lb).				
106	Stick (1/2 cup)-----------	1 stick--------------------	76	16	540	1
107	Tablespoon (about 1/8 stick).	1 tbsp--------------------	9	16	65	Trace
108	Pat (1 1/4 in square, 1/3 in high; 120 per lb).	1 pat---------------------	4	16	25	Trace
109	Fats, cooking (vegetable shortenings).	1 cup---------------------	200	0	1,770	0
110		1 tbsp--------------------	13	0	110	0
111	Lard----------------------------	1 cup---------------------	205	0	1,850	0
112		1 tbsp--------------------	13	0	115	0
	Margarine:				
	Regular (1 brick or 4 sticks per lb):				
113	Stick (1/2 cup)--------------	1 stick--------------------	113	16	815	1
114	Tablespoon (about 1/8 stick)-	1 tbsp--------------------	14	16	100	Trace
115	Pat (1 in square, 1/3 in high; 90 per lb).	1 pat---------------------	5	16	35	Trace
116	Soft, two 8-oz containers per lb.	1 container--------------	227	16	1,635	1
117		1 tbsp--------------------	14	16	100	Trace
	Whipped (6 sticks per lb):				
118	Stick (1/2 cup)--------------	1 stick--------------------	76	16	545	Trace
119	Tablespoon (about 1/8 stick)-	1 tbsp--------------------	9	16	70	Trace

[9]Content of fat, vitamin A, and carbohydrate varies. Consult the label when precise values are needed for special diets.
[10]Applies to product made with milk containing no added vitamin A.
[11]Based on year-round average.
[12]Based on average vitamin A content of fortified margarine. Federal specifications for fortified margarine require a minimum of 15,000 International Units (I.U.) of vitamin A per pound.

Fat	Fatty Acids			Carbo-hydrate	Calcium	Phos-phorus	Iron	Potas-sium	Vitamin A value	Thiamin	Ribo-flavin	Niacin	Ascorbic acid
	Satu-rated (total)	Unsaturated											
		Oleic	Lino-leic										
(F)	(G)	(H)	(I)	(J)	(K)	(L)	(M)	(N)	(O)	(P)	(Q)	(R)	(S)
Grams	Grams	Grams	Grams	Grams	Milli-grams	Milli-grams	Milli-grams	Milli-grams	Inter-national units	Milli-grams	Milli-grams	Milli-grams	Milli-grams
3	1.8	.6	.1	42	343	269	.2	439	[10]120	.08	.40	.2	1
4	2.3	.8	.1	16	415	326	.2	531	[10]150	.10	.49	.3	2
Trace	.3	.1	Trace	17	452	355	.2	579	[10]20	.11	.53	.3	2
7	4.8	1.7	.1	11	274	215	.1	351	280	.07	.32	.2	1
6	1.7	2.0	.6	1	28	90	1.0	65	260	.04	.15	Trace	0
Trace	0	0	0	Trace	4	4	Trace	45	0	Trace	.09	Trace	0
6	1.7	2.1	.6	Trace	26	86	.9	15	310	.04	.07	Trace	0
6	2.4	2.2	.6	1	26	80	.9	58	290	.03	.13	Trace	0
6	1.7	2.0	.6	1	28	90	1.0	65	260	.04	.14	Trace	0
6	1.7	2.0	.6	1	28	90	1.0	65	260	.04	.13	Trace	0
7	2.8	2.3	.6	1	47	97	.9	85	310	.04	.16	Trace	0
92	57.3	23.1	2.1	Trace	27	26	.2	29	[11]3,470	.01	.04	Trace	0
12	7.2	2.9	.3	Trace	3	3	Trace	4	[11]430	Trace	Trace	Trace	0
4	2.5	1.0	.1	Trace	1	1	Trace	1	[11]150	Trace	Trace	Trace	0
61	38.2	15.4	1.4	Trace	18	17	.1	20	[11]2,310	Trace	.03	Trace	0
8	4.7	1.9	.2	Trace	2	2	Trace	2	[11]290	Trace	Trace	Trace	0
3	1.9	.8	.1	Trace	1	1	Trace	1	[11]120	0	Trace	Trace	0
200	48.8	88.2	48.4	0	0	0	0	0	—	0	0	0	0
13	3.2	5.7	3.1	0	0	0	0	0	—	0	0	0	0
205	81.0	83.8	20.5	0	0	0	0	0	0	0	0	0	0
13	5.1	5.3	1.3	0	0	0	0	0	0	0	0	0	0
92	16.7	42.9	24.9	Trace	27	26	.2	29	[12]3,750	.01	.04	Trace	0
12	2.1	5.3	3.1	Trace	3	3	Trace	4	[12]470	Trace	Trace	Trace	0
4	.7	1.9	1.1	Trace	1	1	Trace	1	[12]170	Trace	Trace	Trace	0
184	32.5	71.5	65.4	Trace	53	52	.4	59	[12]7,500	.01	.08	.1	0
12	2.0	4.5	4.1	Trace	3	3	Trace	4	[12]470	Trace	Trace	Trace	0
61	11.2	28.7	16.7	Trace	18	17	.1	20	[12]2,500	Trace	.03	Trace	0
8	1.4	3.6	2.1	Trace	2	2	Trace	2	[12]310	Trace	Trace	Trace	0

NUTRIENTS IN INDICATED QUANTITY

NUTRITIVE VALUES OF THE EDIBLE PART OF FOODS - Continued

(Dashes (—) denote lack of reliable data for a constituent believed to be present in measurable amount)

Item No. (A)	Foods, approximate measures, units, and weight (edible part unless footnotes indicate otherwise) (B)		Water (C)	Food energy (D)	Protein (E)
		Grams	Percent	Calories	Grams

FATS, OILS; RELATED PRODUCTS—Con.

Oils, salad or cooking:

120	Corn-----------------------	1 cup---------------------	218	0	1,925	0
121		1 tbsp--------------------	14	0	120	0
122	Olive-----------------------	1 cup---------------------	216	0	1,910	0
123		1 tbsp--------------------	14	0	120	0
124	Peanut-----------------------	1 cup---------------------	216	0	1,910	0
125		1 tbsp--------------------	14	0	120	0
126	Safflower--------------------	1 cup---------------------	218	0	1,925	0
127		1 tbsp--------------------	14	0	120	0
128	Soybean oil, hydrogenated (partially hardened).	1 cup---------------------	218	0	1,925	0
129		1 tbsp--------------------	14	0	120	0
130	Soybean-cottonseed oil blend, hydrogenated.	1 cup---------------------	218	0	1,925	0
131		1 tbsp--------------------	14	0	120	0
	Salad dressings: Commercial: Blue cheese:					
132	Regular------------------	1 tbsp--------------------	15	32	75	1
133	Low calorie (5 Cal per tsp)	1 tbsp--------------------	16	84	10	Trace
	French:					
134	Regular------------------	1 tbsp--------------------	16	39	65	Trace
135	Low calorie (5 Cal per tsp)	1 tbsp--------------------	16	77	15	Trace
	Italian:					
136	Regular------------------	1 tbsp--------------------	15	28	85	Trace
137	Low calorie (2 Cal per tsp)	1 tbsp--------------------	15	90	10	Trace
138	Mayonnaise------------------	1 tbsp--------------------	14	15	100	Trace
	Mayonnaise type:					
139	Regular------------------	1 tbsp--------------------	15	41	65	Trace
140	Low calorie (8 Cal per tsp)	1 tbsp--------------------	16	81	20	Trace
141	Tartar sauce, regular--------	1 tbsp--------------------	14	34	75	Trace
	Thousand Island:					
142	Regular------------------	1 tbsp--------------------	16	32	80	Trace
143	Low calorie (10 Cal per tsp)	1 tbsp--------------------	15	68	25	Trace
	From home recipe:					
144	Cooked type[13]-----------	1 tbsp--------------------	16	68	25	1

FISH, SHELLFISH, MEAT, POULTRY; RELATED PRODUCTS

Fish and shellfish:

145	Bluefish, baked with butter or margarine.	3 oz----------------------	85	68	135	22
	Clams:					
146	Raw, meat only----------------	3 oz----------------------	85	82	65	11
147	Canned, solids and liquid-----	3 oz----------------------	85	86	45	7
148	Crabmeat (white or king), canned, not pressed down.	1 cup---------------------	135	77	135	24
149	Fish sticks, breaded, cooked, frozen (stick, 4 by 1 by 1/2 in).	1 fish stick or 1 oz-----	28	66	50	5
150	Haddock, breaded, fried[14]-------	3 oz----------------------	85	66	140	17
151	Ocean perch, breaded, fried[14]---	1 fillet-----------------	85	59	195	16
152	Oysters, raw, meat only (13-19 medium Selects).	1 cup--------------------	240	85	160	20
153	Salmon, pink, canned, solids and liquid.	3 oz---------------------	85	71	120	17
154	Sardines, Atlantic, canned in oil, drained solids.	3 oz---------------------	85	62	175	20
155	Scallops, frozen, breaded, fried, reheated.	6 scallops---------------	90	60	175	16
156	Shad, baked with butter or margarine, bacon.	3 oz---------------------	85	64	170	20

[13] Fatty acid values apply to product made with regular-type margarine.
[14] Dipped in egg, milk or water, and breadcrumbs; fried in vegetable shortening.
[15] If bones are discarded, value for calcium will be greatly reduced.

		Fatty Acids											
Fat	Saturated (total)	Unsaturated Oleic	Unsaturated Linoleic	Carbohydrate	Calcium	Phosphorus	Iron	Potassium	Vitamin A value	Thiamin	Riboflavin	Niacin	Ascorbic acid
(F)	(G)	(H)	(I)	(J)	(K)	(L)	(M)	(N)	(O)	(P)	(Q)	(R)	(S)
Grams	Grams	Grams	Grams	Grams	Milligrams	Milligrams	Milligrams	Milligrams	International units	Milligrams	Milligrams	Milligrams	Milligrams
218	27.7	53.6	125.1	0	0	0	0	0	—	0	0	0	0
14	1.7	3.3	7.8	0	0	0	0	0	—	0	0	0	0
216	30.7	154.4	17.7	0	0	0	0	0	—	0	0	0	0
14	1.9	9.7	1.1	0	0	0	0	0	—	0	0	0	0
216	37.4	98.5	67.0	0	0	0	0	0	—	0	0	0	0
14	2.3	6.2	4.2	0	0	0	0	0	—	0	0	0	0
218	20.5	25.9	159.8	0	0	0	0	0	—	0	0	0	0
14	1.3	1.6	10.0	0	0	0	0	0	—	0	0	0	0
218	31.8	93.1	75.6	0	0	0	0	0	—	0	0	0	0
14	2.0	5.8	4.7	0	0	0	0	0	—	0	0	0	0
218	38.2	63.0	99.6	0	0	0	0	0	—	0	0	0	0
14	2.4	3.9	6.2	0	0	0	0	0	—	0	0	0	0
8	1.6	1.7	3.8	1	12	11	Trace	6	30	Trace	.02	Trace	Trace
1	.5	.3	Trace	1	10	8	Trace	5	30	Trace	.01	Trace	Trace
6	1.1	1.3	3.2	3	2	2	.1	13	—	—	—	—	—
1	.1	.1	.4	2	2	2	.1	13	—	—	—	—	—
9	1.6	1.9	4.7	1	2	1	Trace	2	Trace	Trace	Trace	Trace	—
1	.1	.1	.4	Trace	Trace	1	Trace	2	Trace	Trace	Trace	Trace	—
11	2.0	2.4	5.6	Trace	3	4	.1	5	40	Trace	.01	Trace	—
6	1.1	1.4	3.2	2	2	4	Trace	1	30	Trace	Trace	Trace	—
2	.4	.4	1.0	2	3	4	Trace	1	40	Trace	Trace	Trace	—
8	1.5	1.8	4.1	1	3	4	.1	11	30	Trace	Trace	Trace	Trace
8	1.4	1.7	4.0	2	2	3	.1	18	50	Trace	Trace	Trace	Trace
2	.4	.4	1.0	2	2	3	.1	17	50	Trace	Trace	Trace	Trace
2	.5	.6	.3	2	14	15	.1	19	80	.01	.03	Trace	Trace
4	—	—	—	0	25	244	0.6	—	40	0.09	0.08	1.6	—
1	—	—	—	2	59	138	5.2	154	90	.08	.15	1.1	8
1	0.2	Trace	Trace	2	47	116	3.5	119	—	.01	.09	.9	—
3	.6	0.4	0.1	1	61	246	1.1	149	—	.11	.11	2.6	—
3	—	—	—	2	3	47	.1	—	0	.01	.02	.5	—
5	1.4	2.2	1.2	5	34	210	1.0	296	—	.03	.06	2.7	2
11	2.7	4.4	2.3	6	28	192	1.1	242	—	.10	.10	1.6	—
4	1.3	.2	.1	8	226	343	13.2	290	740	.34	.43	6.0	—
5	.9	.8	.1	0	[15]167	243	.7	307	60	.03	.16	6.8	—
9	3.0	2.5	.5	0	372	424	2.5	502	190	.02	.17	4.6	—
8	—	—	—	9	—	—	—	—	—	—	—	—	—
10	—	—	—	0	20	266	.5	320	30	.11	.22	7.3	—

No Milk Today

NUTRITIVE VALUES OF THE EDIBLE PART OF FOODS · Continued

(Dashes (—) denote lack of reliable data for a constituent believed to be present in measurable amount)

Item No. (A)	Foods, approximate measures, units, and weight (edible part unless footnotes indicate otherwise) (B)			Water (C)	Food energy (D)	Pro- tein (E)
			Grams	Per- cent	Cal- ories	Grams

FISH, SHELLFISH, MEAT, POULTRY;
RELATED PRODUCTS—Con.

	Fish and shellfish—Continued Shrimp:					
157	Canned meat-----------------	3 oz-----------------------	85	70	100	21
158	French fried[16]-------------	3 oz-----------------------	85	57	190	17
159	Tuna, canned in oil, drained solids.	3 oz-----------------------	85	61	170	24
160	Tuna salad[17]---------------	1 cup----------------------	205	70	350	30
	Meat and meat products:					
161	Bacon, (20 slices per lb, raw), broiled or fried, crisp.	2 slices-------------------	15	8	85	4
	Beef,[18] cooked: Cuts braised, simmered or pot roasted:					
162	Lean and fat (piece, 2 1/2 by 2 1/2 by 3/4 in)	3 oz-----------------------	85	53	245	23
163	Lean only from item 162-----	2.5 oz---------------------	72	62	140	22
	Ground beef, broiled:					
164	Lean with 10% fat-----------	3 oz or patty 3 by 5/8 in--	85	60	185	23
165	Lean with 21% fat-----------	2.9 oz or patty 3 by 5/8 in	82	54	235	20
	Roast, oven cooked, no liquid added: Relatively fat, such as rib:					
166	Lean and fat (2 pieces, 4 1/8 by 2 1/4 by 1/4 in).	3 oz-----------------------	85	40	375	17
167	Lean only from item 166---	1.8 oz---------------------	51	57	125	14
	Relatively lean, such as heel of round:					
168	Lean and fat (2 pieces, 4 1/8 by 2 1/4 by 1/4 in).	3 oz-----------------------	85	62	165	25
169	Lean only from item 168---	2.8 oz---------------------	78	65	125	24
	Steak: Relatively fat—sirloin, broiled:					
170	Lean and fat (piece, 2 1/2 by 2 1/2 by 3/4 in).	3 oz-----------------------	85	44	330	20
171	Lean only from item 170---	2.0 oz---------------------	56	59	115	18
	Relatively lean—round, braised:					
172	Lean and fat (piece, 4 1/8 by 2 1/4 by 1/2 in).	3 oz-----------------------	85	55	220	24
173	Lean only from item 172---	2.4 oz---------------------	68	61	130	21
	Beef, canned:					
174	Corned beef-----------------	3 oz-----------------------	85	59	185	22
175	Corned beef hash------------	1 cup----------------------	220	67	400	19
176	Beef, dried, chipped--------	2 1/2-oz jar---------------	71	48	145	24
177	Beef and vegetable stew-----	1 cup----------------------	245	82	220	16
178	Beef potpie (home recipe), baked[19] (piece, 1/3 of 9-in diam. pie).	1 piece--------------------	210	55	515	21
179	Chili con carne with beans, canned.	1 cup----------------------	255	72	340	19
180	Chop suey with beef and pork (home recipe).	1 cup----------------------	250	75	300	26
181	Heart, beef, lean, braised------	3 oz-----------------------	85	61	160	27
	Lamb, cooked: Chop, rib (cut 3 per lb with bone), broiled:					
182	Lean and fat----------------	3.1 oz---------------------	89	43	360	18
183	Lean only from item 182-----	2 oz-----------------------	57	60	120	16

[16] Dipped in egg, breadcrumbs, and flour or batter.
[17] Prepared with tuna, celery, salad dressing (mayonnaise type), pickle, onion, and egg.
[18] Outer layer of fat on the cut was removed to within approximately 1/2 in of the lean. Deposits of fat within the cut were not removed.
[19] Crust made with vegetable shortening and enriched flour.

		NUTRIENTS IN INDICATED QUANTITY											
	Fatty Acids												
Fat	Satu- rated (total)	Unsaturated		Carbo- hydrate	Calcium	Phos- phorus	Iron	Potas- sium	Vitamin A value	Thiamin	Ribo- flavin	Niacin	Ascorbic acid
		Oleic	Lino- leic										
(F)	(G)	(H)	(I)	(J)	(K)	(L)	(M)	(N)	(O)	(P)	(Q)	(R)	(S)
Grams	Grams	Grams	Grams	Grams	Milli- grams	Milli- grams	Milli- grams	Milli- grams	Inter- national units	Milli- grams	Milli- grams	Milli- grams	Milli- grams
1	.1	.1	Trace	1	98	224	2.6	104	50	.01	.03	1.5	—
9	2.3	3.7	2.0	9	61	162	1.7	195	—	.03	.07	2.3	—
7	1.7	1.7	.7	0	7	199	1.6	—	70	.04	.10	10.1	—
22	4.3	6.3	6.7	7	41	291	2.7	—	590	.08	.23	10.3	2
8	2.5	3.7	.7	Trace	2	34	.5	35	0	.08	.05	.8	—
16	6.8	6.5	.4	0	10	114	2.9	184	30	.04	.18	3.6	—
5	2.1	1.8	.2	0	10	108	2.7	176	10	.04	.17	3.3	—
10	4.0	3.9	.3	0	10	196	3.0	261	20	.08	.20	5.1	—
17	7.0	6.7	.4	0	9	159	2.6	221	30	.07	.17	4.4	—
33	14.0	13.6	.8	0	8	158	2.2	189	70	.05	.13	3.1	—
7	3.0	2.5	.3	0	6	131	1.8	161	10	.04	.11	2.6	—
7	2.8	2.7	.2	0	11	208	3.2	279	10	.06	.19	4.5	—
3	1.2	1.0	0.1	0	10	199	3.0	268	Trace	0.06	0.18	4.3	—
27	11.3	11.1	.6	0	9	162	2.5	220	50	.05	.15	4.0	—
4	1.8	1.6	.2	0	7	146	2.2	202	10	.05	.14	3.6	—
13	5.5	5.2	.4	0	10	213	3.0	272	20	.07	.19	4.8	—
4	1.7	1.5	.2	0	9	182	2.5	238	10	.05	.16	4.1	—
10	4.9	4.5	.2	0	17	90	3.7	—	—	.01	.20	2.9	—
25	11.9	10.9	.5	24	29	147	4.4	440	—	.02	.20	4.6	—
4	2.1	2.0	.1	0	14	287	3.6	142	—	.05	.23	2.7	0
11	4.9	4.5	.2	15	29	184	2.9	613	2,400	.15	.17	4.7	17
30	7.9	12.8	6.7	39	29	149	3.8	334	1,720	.30	.30	5.5	6
16	7.5	6.8	.3	31	82	321	4.3	594	150	.08	.18	3.3	—
17	8.5	6.2	.7	13	60	248	4.8	425	600	.28	.38	5.0	33
5	1.5	1.1	.6	1	5	154	5.0	197	20	.21	1.04	6.5	1
32	14.8	12.1	1.2	0	8	139	1.0	200	—	.11	.19	4.1	—
6	2.5	2.1	.2	0	6	121	1.1	174	—	.09	.15	3.4	—

NUTRITIVE VALUES OF THE EDIBLE PART OF FOODS · Continued

(Dashes (—) denote lack of reliable data for a constituent believed to be present in measurable amount)

Item No.	Foods, approximate measures, units, and weight (edible part unless footnotes indicate otherwise)		Water	Food energy	Protein
(A)	(B)		(C)	(D)	(E)
		Grams	Percent	Calories	Grams

FISH, SHELLFISH, MEAT, POULTRY;
RELATED PRODUCTS—Con.

Meat and meat products—Continued
Lamb, cooked—Continued
Leg, roasted:

Item No.	Food	Measure	Grams	Percent	Calories	Grams
184	Lean and fat (2 pieces, 4 1/8 by 2 1/4 by 1/4 in).	3 oz	85	54	235	22
185	Lean only from item 184	2.5 oz	71	62	130	20
	Shoulder, roasted:					
186	Lean and fat (3 pieces, 2 1/2 by 2 1/2 by 1/4 in).	3 oz	85	50	285	18
187	Lean only from item 186	2.3 oz	64	61	130	17
188	Liver, beef, fried[20] (slice, 6 1/2 by 2 3/8 by 3/8 in).	3 oz	85	56	195	22
	Pork, cured, cooked:					
189	Ham, light cure, lean and fat, roasted (2 pieces, 4 1/8 by 2 1/4 by 1/4 in).[22]	3 oz	85	54	245	18
	Luncheon meat:					
190	Boiled ham, slice (8 per 8-oz pkg.).	1 oz	28	59	65	5
	Canned, spiced or unspiced:					
191	Slice, approx. 3 by 2 by 1/2 in.	1 slice	60	55	175	9
	Pork, fresh,[18] cooked: Chop, loin (cut 3 per lb with bone), broiled:					
192	Lean and fat	2.7 oz	78	42	305	19
193	Lean only from item 192	2 oz	56	53	150	17
	Roast, oven cooked, no liquid added:					
194	Lean and fat (piece, 2 1/2 by 2 1/2 by 3/4 in).	3 oz	85	46	310	21
195	Lean only from item 194	2.4 oz	68	55	175	20
	Shoulder cut, simmered:					
196	Lean and fat (3 pieces, 2 1/2 by 2 1/2 by 1/4 in).	3 oz	85	46	320	20
197	Lean only from item 196	2.2 oz	63	60	135	18
	Sausages (see also Luncheon meat (items 190-191)):					
198	Bologna, slice (8 per 8-oz pkg.).	1 slice	28	56	85	3
199	Braunschweiger, slice (6 per 6-oz pkg.).	1 slice	28	53	90	4
200	Brown and serve (10-11 per 8-oz pkg.), browned.	1 link	17	40	70	3
201	Deviled ham, canned	1 tbsp	13	51	45	2
202	Frankfurter (8 per 1-lb pkg.), cooked (reheated).	1 frankfurter	56	57	170	7
203	Meat, potted (beef, chicken, turkey), canned.	1 tbsp	13	61	30	2
204	Pork link (16 per 1-lb pkg.), cooked.	1 link	13	35	60	2
	Salami:					
205	Dry type, slice (12 per 4-oz pkg.).	1 slice	10	30	45	2
206	Cooked type, slice (8 per 8-oz pkg.).	1 slice	28	51	90	5
207	Vienna sausage (7 per 4-oz can).	1 sausage	16	63	40	2

[18] Outer layer of fat on the cut was removed to within approximately 1/2 in of the lean. Deposits of fat within the cut were not removed.
[20] Regular-type margarine used.
[21] Value varies widely.
[22] About one-fourth of the outer layer of fat on the cut was removed. Deposits of fat within the cut were not removed.

Fat	Fatty Acids			Carbo-hydrate	Calcium	Phos-phorus	Iron	Potas-sium	Vitamin A value	Thiamin	Ribo-flavin	Niacin	Ascorbic acid
	Satu-rated (total)	Unsaturated											
		Oleic	Lino-leic										
(F)	(G)	(H)	(I)	(J)	(K)	(L)	(M)	(N)	(O)	(P)	(Q)	(R)	(S)
Grams	Grams	Grams	Grams	Grams	Milli-grams	Milli-grams	Milli-grams	Milli-grams	Inter-national units	Milli-grams	Milli-grams	Milli-grams	Milli-grams
16	7.3	6.0	.6	0	9	177	1.4	241	—	.13	.23	4.7	—
5	2.1	1.8	.2	0	9	169	1.4	227	—	.12	.21	4.4	—
23	10.8	8.8	.9	0	9	146	1.0	206	—	.11	.20	4.0	—
6	3.6	2.3	.2	0	8	140	1.0	193	—	.10	.18	3.7	—
9	2.5	3.5	.9	5	9	405	7.5	323	[21]45,390	.22	3.56	14.0	23
19	6.8	7.9	1.7	0	8	146	2.2	199	0	.40	.15	3.1	—
5	1.7	2.0	.4	0	3	47	.8	—	0	.12	.04	.7	—
15	5.4	6.7	1.0	1	5	65	1.3	133	0	.19	.13	1.8	—
25	8.9	10.4	2.2	0	9	209	2.7	216	0	0.75	0.22	4.5	—
9	3.1	3.6	.8	0	7	181	2.2	192	0	.63	.18	3.8	—
24	8.7	10.2	2.2	0	9	218	2.7	233	0	.78	.22	4.8	—
10	3.5	4.1	.8	0	9	211	2.6	224	0	.73	.21	4.4	—
26	9.3	10.9	2.3	0	9	118	2.6	158	0	.46	.21	4.1	—
6	2.2	2.6	.6	0	8	111	2.3	146	0	.42	.19	3.7	—
8	3.0	3.4	.5	Trace	2	36	.5	65	—	.05	.06	.7	—
8	2.6	3.4	.8	1	3	69	1.7	—	1,850	.05	.41	2.3	—
6	2.3	2.8	.7	Trace	—	—	—	—	—	—	—	—	—
4	1.5	1.8	.4	0	1	12	.3	—	0	.02	.01	.2	—
15	5.6	6.5	1.2	1	3	57	.8	—	—	.08	.11	1.4	—
2	—	—	—	0	—	—	—	—	—	Trace	.03	.2	—
6	2.1	2.4	.5	Trace	1	21	.3	35	0	.10	.04	.5	—
4	1.6	1.6	.1	Trace	1	28	.4	—	—	.04	.03	.5	—
7	3.1	3.0	.2	Trace	3	57	.7	—	—	.07	.07	1.2	—
3	1.2	1.4	.2	Trace	1	24	.3	—	—	.01	.02	.4	—

NUTRITIVE VALUES OF THE EDIBLE PART OF FOODS - Continued

(Dashes (—) denote lack of reliable data for a constituent believed to be present in measurable amount)

Item No. (A)	Foods, approximate measures, units, and weight (edible part unless footnotes indicate otherwise) (B)		Water (C)	Food energy (D)	Protein (E)
			Grams	Percent	Calories	Grams

FISH, SHELLFISH, MEAT, POULTRY; RELATED PRODUCTS—Con.

Meat and meat products—Continued
Veal, medium fat, cooked, bone removed:

208	Cutlet (4 1/8 by 2 1/4 by 1/2 in), braised or broiled.	3 oz-------------------	85	60	185	23
209	Rib (2 pieces, 4 1/8 by 2 1/4 by 1/4 in), roasted.	3 oz-------------------	85	55	230	23

Poultry and poultry products:
Chicken, cooked:

210	Breast, fried,[23] bones removed, 1/2 breast (3.3 oz with bones).	2.8 oz-----------------	79	58	160	26
211	Drumstick, fried,[23] bones removed (2 oz with bones).	1.3 oz-----------------	38	55	90	12
212	Half broiler, broiled, bones removed (10.4 oz with bones).	6.2 oz-----------------	176	71	240	42
213	Chicken, canned, boneless-------	3 oz-------------------	85	65	170	18
214	Chicken a la king, cooked (home recipe).	1 cup------------------	245	68	470	27
215	Chicken and noodles, cooked (home recipe).	1 cup------------------	240	71	365	22

Chicken chow mein:

216	Canned------------------------	1 cup------------------	250	89	95	7
217	From home recipe--------------	1 cup------------------	250	78	255	31
218	Chicken potpie (home recipe), baked,[19] piece (1/3 or 9-in diam. pie).	1 piece----------------	232	57	545	23

Turkey, roasted, flesh without skin:

219	Dark meat, piece, 2 1/2 by 1 5/8 by 1/4 in.	4 pieces---------------	85	61	175	26
220	Light meat, piece, 4 by 2 by 1/4 in.	2 pieces---------------	85	62	150	28

Light and dark meat:

221	Chopped or diced------------	1 cup------------------	140	61	265	44
222	Pieces (1 slice white meat, 4 by 2 by 1/4 in with 2 slices dark meat, 2 1/2 by 1 5/8 by 1/4 in).	3 pieces---------------	85	61	160	27

FRUITS AND FRUIT PRODUCTS

Apples, raw, unpeeled, without cores:

223	2 3/4-in diam. (about 3 per lb with cores).	1 apple-----------------	138	84	80	Trace
224	3 1/4 in diam. (about 2 per lb with cores).	1 apple-----------------	212	84	125	Trace
225	Applejuice, bottled or canned[24]---	1 cup--------------------	248	88	120	Trace

Applesauce, canned:

226	Sweetened---------------------	1 cup------------------	255	76	230	1
227	Unsweetened-------------------	1 cup------------------	244	89	100	Trace

Apricots:

228	Raw, without pits (about 12 per lb with pits).	3 apricots--------------	107	85	55	1
229	Canned in heavy sirup (halves and sirup).	1 cup-------------------	258	77	220	2

Dried:

230	Uncooked (28 large or 37 medium halves per cup).	1 cup-------------------	130	25	340	7

[19] Crust made with vegetable shortening and enriched flour.
[23] Vegetable shortening used.
[24] Also applies to pasteurized apple cider.
[25] Applies to product without added ascorbic acid. For value of product with added ascorbic acid, refer to label.

		Fatty Acids											
Fat	Satu-rated (total)	Unsaturated Oleic	Unsaturated Lino-leic	Carbo-hydrate	Calcium	Phos-phorus	Iron	Potas-sium	Vitamin A value	Thiamin	Ribo-flavin	Niacin	Ascorbic acid
(F)	(G)	(H)	(I)	(J)	(K)	(L)	(M)	(N)	(O)	(P)	(Q)	(R)	(S)
Grams	Grams	Grams	Grams	Grams	Milli-grams	Milli-grams	Milli-grams	Milli-grams	Inter-national units	Milli-grams	Milli-grams	Milli-grams	Milli-grams
9	4.0	3.4	.4	0	9	196	2.7	258	—	.06	.21	4.6	—
14	6.1	5.1	.6	0	10	211	2.9	259	—	.11	.26	6.6	—
5	1.4	1.8	1.1	1	9	218	1.3	—	70	.04	.17	11.6	—
4	1.1	1.3	.9	Trace	6	89	.9	—	50	.03	.15	2.7	—
7	2.2	2.5	1.3	0	16	355	3.0	483	160	.09	.34	15.5	—
10	3.2	3.8	2.0	0	18	210	1.3	117	200	.03	.11	3.7	3
34	2.7	14.3	3.3	12	127	358	2.5	404	1,130	.10	.42	5.4	12
18	5.9	7.1	3.5	26	26	247	2.2	149	430	.05	.17	4.3	Trace
Trace	—	—	—	18	45	35	1.3	418	150	0.05	0.10	1.0	13
10	2.4	3.4	3.1	10	58	293	2.5	473	280	.08	.23	4.3	10
31	11.3	10.9	5.6	42	70	232	3.0	343	3,090	.34	.31	5.5	5
7	2.1	1.5	1.5	0	—	—	2.0	338	—	.03	.20	3.6	—
3	.9	.6	.7	0	—	—	1.0	349	—	.04	.12	9.4	—
9	2.5	1.7	1.8	0	11	351	2.5	514	—	.07	.25	10.8	—
5	1.5	1.0	1.1	0	7	213	1.5	312	—	.04	.15	6.5	—
1	—	—	—	20	10	14	.4	152	120	.04	.03	.1	6
1	—	—	—	31	15	21	.6	233	190	.06	.04	.2	8
Trace	—	—	—	30	15	22	1.5	250	—	.02	.05	.2	[25]2
Trace	—	—	—	61	10	13	1.3	166	100	.05	.03	.1	[25]3
Trace	—	—	—	26	10	12	1.2	190	100	.05	.02	.1	[25]2
Trace	—	—	—	14	18	25	.5	301	2,890	.03	.04	.6	11
Trace	—	—	—	57	28	39	.8	604	4,490	.05	.05	1.0	10
1	—	—	—	86	87	140	7.2	1,273	14,170	.01	.21	4.3	16

NUTRITIVE VALUES OF THE EDIBLE PART OF FOODS · Continued

(Dashes (—) denote lack of reliable data for a constituent believed to be present in measurable amount)

Item No. (A)	Foods, approximate measures, units, and weight (edible part unless footnotes indicate otherwise) (B)		Water (C)	Food energy (D)	Pro-tein (E)
		Grams	Per-cent	Cal-ories	Grams

FRUITS AND FRUIT PRODUCTS—Con.

	Apricots—Continued				
	Dried—Continued				
231	Cooked, unsweetened, fruit and liquid.	1 cup---------------------- 250	76	215	4
232	Apricot nectar, canned------------	1 cup---------------------- 251	85	145	1
	Avocados, raw, whole, without skins and seeds:				
233	California, mid- and late-winter (with skin and seed, 3 1/8-in diam.; wt., 10 oz).	1 avocado------------------ 216	74	370	5
234	Florida, late summer and fall (with skin and seed, 3 5/8-in diam.; wt., 1 lb).	1 avocado------------------ 304	78	390	4
235	Banana without peel (about 2.6 per lb with peel).	1 banana------------------- 119	76	100	1
236	Banana flakes---------------------	1 tbsp---------------------- 6	3	20	Trace
237	Blackberries, raw-----------------	1 cup---------------------- 144	85	85	2
238	Blueberries, raw------------------	1 cup---------------------- 145	83	90	1
	Cantaloup. See Muskmelons (item 271).				
	Cherries:				
239	Sour (tart), red, pitted, can-ned, water pack.	1 cup---------------------- 244	88	105	2
240	Sweet, raw, without pits and stems.	10 cherries---------------- 68	80	45	1
241	Cranberry juice cocktail, bottled, sweetened.	1 cup---------------------- 253	83	165	Trace
242	Cranberry sauce, sweetened, canned, strained.	1 cup---------------------- 277	62	405	Trace
	Dates:				
243	Whole, without pits-------------	10 dates------------------- 80	23	220	2
244	Chopped-------------------------	1 cup---------------------- 178	23	490	4
245	Fruit cocktail, canned, in heavy sirup.	1 cup---------------------- 255	80	195	1
	Grapefruit:				
	Raw, medium, 3 3/4-in diam. (about 1 lb 1 oz):				
246	Pink or red--------------------	1/2 grapefruit with peel[28] 241	89	50	1
247	White--------------------------	1/2 grapefruit with peel[28] 241	89	45	1
248	Canned, sections with sirup-----	1 cup---------------------- 254	81	180	2
	Grapefruit juice:				
249	Raw, pink, red, or white--------	1 cup---------------------- 246	90	95	1
	Canned, white:				
250	Unsweetened-------------------	1 cup---------------------- 247	89	100	1 *
251	Sweetened---------------------	1 cup---------------------- 250	86	135	1
	Frozen, concentrate, unsweetened:				
252	Undiluted, 6-fl oz can---------	1 can---------------------- 207	62	300	4
253	Diluted with 3 parts water by volume.	1 cup---------------------- 247	89	100	1
254	Dehydrated crystals, prepared with water (1 lb yields about 1 gal).	1 cup---------------------- 247	90	100	1
	Grapes, European type (adherent skin), raw:				
255	Thompson Seedless---------------	10 grapes------------------ 50	81	35	Trace
256	Tokay and Emperor, seeded types-	10 grapes[30]-------------- 60	81	40	Trace

[26] Based on product with label claim of 45% of U.S. RDA in 6 fl oz.
[27] Based on product with label claim of 100% of U.S. RDA in 6 fl oz.
[28] Weight includes peel and membranes between sections. Without these parts, the weight of the edible portion is 123 g for item 246 and 118 g for item 247.
[29] For white-fleshed varieties, value is about 20 International Units (I.U.) per cup; for red-fleshed varieties, 1,080 I.U.
[30] Weight includes seeds. Without seeds, the weight of the edible portion is 57 g.

Fat	Satu-rated (total)	Unsaturated		Carbo-hydrate	Calcium	Phos-phorus	Iron	Potas-sium	Vitamin A value	Thiamin	Ribo-flavin	Niacin	Ascorbic acid
		Oleic	Lino-leic										
(F)	(G)	(H)	(I)	(J)	(K)	(L)	(M)	(N)	(O)	(P)	(Q)	(R)	(S)
Grams	Grams	Grams	Grams	Grams	Milli-grams	Milli-grams	Milli-grams	Milli-grams	Inter-national units	Milli-grams	Milli-grams	Milli-grams	Milli-grams
1	—	—	—	54	55	88	4.5	795	7,500	.01	.13	2.5	8
Trace	—	—	—	37	23	30	.5	379	2,380	.03	.03	.5	[26]36
37	5.5	22.0	3.7	13	22	91	1.3	1,303	630	.24	.43	3.5	30
33	6.7	15.7	5.3	27	30	128	1.8	1,836	880	.33	.61	4.9	43
Trace	—	—	—	26	10	31	.8	440	230	.06	.07	.8	12
Trace	—	—	—	5	2	6	.2	92	50	.01	.01	.2	Trace
1	—	—	—	19	46	27	1.3	245	290	0.04	0.06	0.6	30
1	—	—	—	22	22	19	1.5	117	150	.04	.09	.7	20
Trace	—	—	—	26	37	32	.7	317	1,660	.07	.05	.5	12
Trace	—	—	—	12	15	13	.3	129	70	.03	.04	.3	7
Trace	—	—	—	42	13	8	.8	25	Trace	.03	.03	.1	[27]81
1	—	—	—	104	17	11	.6	83	60	.03	.03	.1	6
Trace	—	—	—	58	47	50	2.4	518	40	.07	.08	1.8	0
1	—	—	—	130	105	112	5.3	1,153	90	.16	.18	3.9	0
Trace	—	—	—	50	23	31	1.0	411	360	.05	.03	1.0	5
Trace	—	—	—	13	20	20	.5	166	540	.05	.02	.2	44
Trace	—	—	—	12	19	19	.5	159	10	.05	.02	.2	44
Trace	—	—	—	45	33	36	.8	343	30	.08	.05	.5	76
Trace	—	—	—	23	22	37	.5	399	([29])	.10	.05	.5	93
Trace	—	—	—	24	20	35	1.0	400	20	.07	.05	.5	84
Trace	—	—	—	32	20	35	1.0	405	30	.08	.05	.5	78
1	—	—	—	72	70	124	.8	1,250	60	.29	.12	1.4	286
Trace	—	—	—	24	25	42	.2	420	20	.10	.04	.5	96
Trace	—	—	—	24	22	40	.2	412	20	.10	.05	.5	91
Trace	—	—	—	9	6	10	.2	87	50	.03	.02	.2	2
Trace	—	—	—	10	7	11	.2	99	60	.03	.02	.2	2

NUTRITIVE VALUES OF THE EDIBLE PART OF FOODS · Continued

(Dashes (—) denote lack of reliable data for a constituent believed to be present in measurable amount)

Item No. (A)	Foods, approximate measures, units, and weight (edible part unless footnotes indicate otherwise) (B)		Water (C)	Food energy (D)	Pro- tein (E)
			Grams	Per- cent	Cal- ories	Grams

FRUITS AND FRUIT PRODUCTS—Con.

Item No.	Foods	Measure	Grams	Water Percent	Food energy Calories	Protein Grams
	Grapejuice:					
257	Canned or bottled-------------	1 cup-----------------	253	83	165	1
	Frozen concentrate, sweetened:					
258	Undiluted, 6-fl oz can--------	1 can-----------------	216	53	395	1
259	Diluted with 3 parts water by volume.	1 cup-----------------	250	86	135	1
260	Grape drink, canned-----------	1 cup-----------------	250	86	135	Trace
261	Lemon, raw, size 165, without peel and seeds (about 4 per lb with peels and seeds).	1 lemon---------------	74	90	20	1
	Lemon juice:					
262	Raw--------------------------	1 cup-----------------	244	91	60	1
263	Canned, or bottled, unsweetened-	1 cup-----------------	244	92	55	1
264	Frozen, single strength, un- sweetened, 6-fl oz can.	1 can-----------------	183	92	40	1
	Lemonade concentrate, frozen:					
265	Undiluted, 6-fl oz can--------	1 can-----------------	219	49	425	Trace
266	Diluted with 4 1/3 parts water by volume.	1 cup-----------------	248	89	105	Trace
	Limeade concentrate, frozen:					
267	Undiluted, 6-fl oz can--------	1 can-----------------	218	50	410	Trace
268	Diluted with 4 1/3 parts water by volume.	1 cup-----------------	247	89	100	Trace
	Limejuice:					
269	Raw--------------------------	1 cup-----------------	246	90	65	1
270	Canned, unsweetened----------	1 cup-----------------	246	90	65	1
	Muskmelons, raw, with rind, with- out seed cavity:					
271	Cantaloup, orange-fleshed (with rind and seed cavity, 5-in diam., 2 1/3 lb).	1/2 melon with rind[33]-----	477	91	80	2
272	Honeydew (with rind and seed cavity, 6 1/2-in diam., 5 1/4 lb).	1/10 melon with rind[33]----	226	91	50	1
	Oranges, all commercial varieties, raw:					
273	Whole, 2 5/8-in diam., without peel and seeds (about 2 1/2 per lb with peel and seeds).	1 orange--------------	131	86	65	1
274	Sections without membranes------	1 cup-----------------	180	86	90	2
	Orange juice:					
275	Raw, all varieties-----------	1 cup-----------------	248	88	110	2
276	Canned, unsweetened-----------	1 cup-----------------	249	87	120	2
	Frozen concentrate:					
277	Undiluted, 6-fl oz can--------	1 can-----------------	213	55	360	5
278	Diluted with 3 parts water by volume.	1 cup-----------------	249	87	120	2
279	Dehydrated crystals, prepared with water (1 lb yields about 1 gal).	1 cup-----------------	248	88	115	1
	Orange and grapefruit juice: Frozen concentrate:					
280	Undiluted, 6-fl oz can--------	1 can-----------------	210	59	330	4
281	Diluted with 3 parts water by volume.	1 cup-----------------	248	88	110	1
282	Papayas, raw, 1/2-in cubes--------	1 cup-----------------	140	89	55	1

[25] Applies to product without added ascorbic acid. For value of product with added ascorbic acid, refer to label.

[31] Applies to product without added ascorbic acid. With added ascorbic acid, based on claim that 6 fl oz of reconstituted juice contain 45% or 50% of the U.S. RDA, value in milligrams is 108 or 120 for a 6-fl oz can (item 258), 36 or 40 for 1 cup of diluted juice (item 259).

[32] For products with added thiamin and riboflavin but without added ascorbic acid, values in milligrams would be 0.60 for thiamin, 0.80 for riboflavin, and trace for ascorbic acid. For products with only ascorbic acid added, value varies with the brand. Consult the label.

[33] Weight includes rind. Without rind, the weight of the edible portion is 272 g for item 271 and 149 g for item 272.

Fat	Saturated (total)	Unsaturated Oleic	Lino leic	Carbohydrate	Calcium	Phosphorus	Iron	Potassium	Vitamin A value	Thiamin	Riboflavin	Niacin	Ascorbic acid
(F)	(G)	(H)	(I)	(J)	(K)	(L)	(M)	(N)	(O)	(P)	(Q)	(R)	(S)
Grams	Grams	Grams	Grams	Grams	Milligrams	Milligrams	Milligrams	Milligrams	International units	Milligrams	Milligrams	Milligrams	Milligrams
Trace	—	—	—	42	28	30	.8	293	—	.10	.05	.5	[25]Trace
Trace	—	—	—	100	22	32	.9	255	40	.13	.22	1.5	[31]32
Trace	—	—	—	33	8	10	.3	85	10	.05	.08	.5	[31]10
Trace	—	—	—	35	8	10	.3	88	—	[32].03	[32].03	.3	([32])
Trace	—	—	—	6	19	12	.4	102	10	.03	.01	.1	39
Trace	—	—	—	20	17	24	.5	344	50	.07	.02	.2	112
Trace	—	—	—	19	17	24	.5	344	50	.07	.02	.2	102
Trace	—	—	—	13	13	16	.5	258	40	.05	.02	.2	81
Trace	—	—	—	112	9	13	.4	153	40	.05	.06	.7	66
Trace	—	—	—	28	2	3	.1	40	10	.01	.02	.2	17
Trace	—	—	—	108	11	13	0.2	129	Trace	0.02	0.02	0.2	26
Trace	—	—	—	27	3	3	Trace	32	Trace	Trace	Trace	Trace	6
Trace	—	—	—	22	22	27	.5	256	20	.05	.02	.2	79
Trace	—	—	—	22	22	27	.5	256	20	.05	.02	.2	52
Trace	—	—	—	20	38	44	1.1	682	9,240	.11	.08	1.6	90
Trace	—	—	—	11	21	24	.6	374	60	.06	.04	.9	34
Trace	—	—	—	16	54	26	.5	263	260	.13	.05	.5	66
Trace	—	—	—	22	74	36	.7	360	360	.18	.07	.7	90
Trace	—	—	—	26	27	42	.5	496	500	.22	.07	1.0	124
Trace	—	—	—	28	25	45	1.0	496	500	.17	.05	.7	100
Trace	—	—	—	87	75	126	.9	1,500	1,620	.68	.11	2.8	360
Trace	—	—	—	29	25	42	.2	503	540	.23	.03	.9	120
Trace	—	—	—	27	25	40	.5	518	500	.20	.07	1.0	109
1	—	—	—	78	61	99	.8	1,308	800	.48	.06	2.3	302
Trace	—	—	—	26	20	32	.2	439	270	.15	.02	.7	102
Trace	—	—	—	14	28	22	.4	328	2,450	.06	.06	.4	78

NUTRITIVE VALUES OF THE EDIBLE PART OF FOODS · Continued

(Dashes (−) denote lack of reliable data for a constituent believed to be present in measurable amount)

Item No. (A)	Foods, approximate measures, units, and weight (edible part unless footnotes indicate otherwise) (B)		Water (C)	Food energy (D)	Protein (E)
		Grams	Per-cent	Cal-ories	Grams
	FRUITS AND FRUIT PRODUCTS –Con.				
	Peaches:				
	Raw:				
283	Whole, 2 1/2-in diam., peeled, pitted (about 4 per lb with peels and pits).	1 peach-----------------	100	89	40	1
284	Sliced------------------------	1 cup--------------------	170	89	65	1
	Canned, yellow-fleshed, solids and liquid (halves or slices):				
285	Sirup pack---------------------	1 cup--------------------	256	79	200	1
286	Water pack---------------------	1 cup--------------------	244	91	75	1
	Dried:				
287	Uncooked-----------------------	1 cup--------------------	160	25	420	5
288	Cooked, unsweetened, halves and juice.	1 cup--------------------	250	77	205	3
	Frozen, sliced, sweetened:				
289	10-oz container----------------	1 container-------------	284	77	250	1
290	Cup----------------------------	1 cup--------------------	250	77	220	1
	Pears:				
	Raw, with skin, cored:				
291	Bartlett, 2 1/2-in diam. (about 2 1/2 per lb with cores and stems).	1 pear-------------------	164	83	100	1
292	Bosc, 2 1/2-in diam. (about 3 per lb with cores and stems).	1 pear-------------------	141	83	85	1
293	D'Anjou, 3-in diam. (about 2 per lb with cores and stems).	1 pear-------------------	200	83	120	1
294	Canned, solids and liquid, sirup pack, heavy (halves or slices).	1 cup--------------------	255	80	195	1
	Pineapple:				
295	Raw, diced--------------------	1 cup--------------------	155	85	80	1
	Canned, heavy sirup pack, solids and liquid:				
296	Crushed, chunks, tidbits-------	1 cup--------------------	255	80	190	1
	Slices and liquid:				
297	Large------------------------	1 slice; 2 1/4 tbsp liquid.	105	80	80	Trace
298	Medium-----------------------	1 slice; 1 1/4 tbsp liquid.	58	80	45	Trace
299	Pineapple juice, unsweetened, canned.	1 cup--------------------	250	86	140	1
	Plums:				
	Raw, without pits:				
300	Japanese and hybrid (2 1/8-in diam., about 6 1/2 per lb with pits).	1 plum-------------------	66	87	30	Trace
301	Prune-type (1 1/2-in diam., about 15 per lb with pits).	1 plum-------------------	28	79	20	Trace
	Canned, heavy sirup pack (Italian prunes), with pits and liquid:				
302	Cup----------------------------	1 cup[36]-----------------	272	77	215	1
303	Portion------------------------	3 plums; 2 3/4 tbsp liquid.[36]	140	77	110	1
	Prunes, dried, "softenized," with pits:				
304	Uncooked-----------------------	4 extra large or 5 large prunes.[36]	49	28	110	1
305	Cooked, unsweetened, all sizes, fruit and liquid.	1 cup[36]-----------------	250	66	255	2

[27]Based on product with label claim of 100% of U.S. RDA in 6 fl oz.
[34]Represents yellow-fleshed varieties. For white-fleshed varieties, value is 50 International Units (I.U.) for 1 peach, 90 I.U. for 1 cup of slices.
[35]Value represents products with added ascorbic acid. For products without added ascorbic acid, value in milligrams is 116 for a 10-oz container, 103 for 1 cup.
[36]Weight includes pits. After removal of the pits, the weight of the edible portion is 258 g for item 302, 133 g for item 303, 43 g for item 304, and 213 g for item 305.

		Fatty Acids											
			Unsaturated										
Fat	Saturated (total)	Oleic	Linoleic	Carbohydrate	Calcium	Phosphorus	Iron	Potassium	Vitamin A value	Thiamin	Riboflavin	Niacin	Ascorbic acid
(F)	(G)	(H)	(I)	(J)	(K)	(L)	(M)	(N)	(O)	(P)	(Q)	(R)	(S)
Grams	Grams	Grams	Grams	Grams	Milligrams	Milligrams	Milligrams	Milligrams	International units	Milligrams	Milligrams	Milligrams	Milligrams
Trace	—	—	—	10	9	19	.5	202	[34]1,330	.02	.05	1.0	7
Trace	—	—	—	16	15	32	.9	343	[34]2,260	.03	.09	1.7	12
Trace	—	—	—	51	10	31	.8	333	1,100	.03	.05	1.5	8
Trace	—	—	—	20	10	32	.7	334	1,100	.02	.07	1.5	7
1	—	—	—	109	77	187	9.6	1,520	6,240	.02	.30	8.5	29
1	—	—	—	54	38	93	4.8	743	3,050	.01	.15	3.8	5
Trace	—	—	—	64	11	37	1.4	352	1,850	0.03	0.11	2.0	[35]116
Trace	—	—	—	57	10	33	1.3	310	1,630	.03	.10	1.8	[35]103
1	—	—	—	25	13	18	.5	213	30	.03	.07	.2	7
1	—	—	—	22	11	16	.4	83	30	.03	.06	.1	6
1	—	—	—	31	16	22	.6	260	40	.04	.08	.2	8
1	—	—	—	50	13	18	.5	214	10	.03	.05	.3	3
Trace	—	—	—	21	26	12	.8	226	110	.14	.05	.3	26
Trace	—	—	—	49	28	13	.8	245	130	.20	.05	.5	18
Trace	—	—	—	20	12	5	.3	101	50	.08	.02	.2	7
Trace	—	—	—	11	6	3	.2	56	30	.05	.01	.1	4
Trace	—	—	—	34	38	23	.8	373	130	.13	.05	.5	[27]80
Trace	—	—	—	8	8	12	.3	112	160	.02	.02	.3	4
Trace	—	—	—	6	3	5	.1	48	80	.01	.01	.1	1
Trace	—	—	—	56	23	26	2.3	367	3,130	.05	.05	1.0	5
Trace	—	—	—	29	12	13	1.2	189	1,610	.03	.03	.5	3
Trace	—	—	—	29	22	34	1.7	298	690	.04	.07	.7	1
1	—	—	—	67	51	79	3.8	695	1,590	.07	.15	1.5	2

NUTRITIVE VALUES OF THE EDIBLE PART OF FOODS · Continued

(Dashes (−) denote lack of reliable data for a constituent believed to be present in measurable amount)

Item No. (A)	Foods, approximate measures, units, and weight (edible part unless footnotes indicate otherwise) (B)		Water (C)	Food energy (D)	Pro-tein (E)
		Grams	Per-cent	Cal-ories	Grams

FRUITS AND FRUIT PRODUCTS—Con.

Item No.	Foods	Measure	Grams	Water	Cal	Protein
306	Prune juice, canned or bottled-----	1 cup--------------------	256	80	195	1
	Raisins, seedless:					
307	Cup, not pressed down------------	1 cup--------------------	145	18	420	4
308	Packet, 1/2 oz (1 1/2 tbsp)------	1 packet-----------------	14	18	40	Trace
	Raspberries, red:					
309	Raw, capped, whole---------------	1 cup--------------------	123	84	70	1
310	Frozen, sweetened, 10-oz container	1 container-------------	284	74	280	2
	Rhubarb, cooked, added sugar:					
311	From raw---;--------------------	1 cup--------------------	270	63	380	1
312	From frozen, sweetened-----------	1 cup--------------------	270	63	385	1
	Strawberries:					
313	Raw, whole berries, capped-----	1 cup--------------------	149	90	55	1
	Frozen, sweetened:					
314	Sliced, 10-oz container------	1 container-------------	284	71	310	1
315	Whole, 1-lb container (about 1 3/4 cups).	1 container-------------	454	76	415	2
316	Tangerine, raw, 2 3/8-in diam., size 176, without peel (about 4 per lb with peels and seeds).	1 tangerine-------------	86	87	40	1
317	Tangerine juice, canned, sweetened.	1 cup--------------------	249	87	125	1
318	Watermelon, raw, 4 by 8 in wedge with rind and seeds (1/16 of 32 2/3-lb melon, 10 by 16 in).	1 wedge with rind and seeds[37]	926	93	110	2

GRAIN PRODUCTS

Item No.	Foods	Measure	Grams	Water	Cal	Protein
	Bagel, 3-in diam.:					
319	Egg---------------------------	1 bagel-----------------	55	32	165	6
320	Water-------------------------	1 bagel-----------------	55	29	165	6
321	Barley, pearled, light, uncooked-	1 cup--------------------	200	11	700	16
	Biscuits, baking powder, 2-in diam. (enriched flour, vegetable shortening):					
322	From home recipe---------------	1 biscuit---------------	28	27	105	2
323	From mix-----------------------	1 biscuit---------------	28	29	90	2
	Breadcrumbs (enriched):[38]					
324	Dry, grated---------------------	1 cup--------------------	100	7	390	13
	Soft. See White bread (items 349-350).					
	Breads:					
325	Boston brown bread, canned, slice, 3 1/4 by 1/2 in.[38]	1 slice-----------------	45	45	95	2
	Cracked-wheat bread (3/4 enriched wheat flour, 1/4 cracked wheat):[38]					
326	Loaf, 1 lb--------------------	1 loaf------------------	454	35	1,195	39
327	Slice (18 per loaf)----------	1 slice-----------------	25	35	65	2
	French or vienna bread, enriched:[38]					
328	Loaf, 1 lb-------------------	1 loaf------------------	454	31	1,315	41
	Slice:					
329	French (5 by 2 1/2 by 1 in)	1 slice-----------------	35	31	100	3
330	Vienna (4 3/4 by 4 by 1/2 in).	1 slice-----------------	25	31	75	2
	Italian bread, enriched:					
331	Loaf, 1 lb-------------------	1 loaf------------------	454	32	1,250	41
332	Slice, 4 1/2 by 3 1/4 by 3/4 in.	1 slice-----------------	30	32	85	3

[37]Weight includes rind and seeds. Without rind and seeds, weight of the edible portion is 426 g.
[38]Made with vegetable shortening.
[39]Applies to product made with white cornmeal. With yellow cornmeal, value is 30 International Units (I.U.).

Fat (F)	Fatty Acids Saturated (total) (G)	Unsaturated Oleic (H)	Lino- leic (I)	Carbo- hydrate (J)	Calcium (K)	Phos- phorus (L)	Iron (M)	Potas- sium (N)	Vitamin A value (O)	Thiamin (P)	Ribo- flavin (Q)	Niacin (R)	Ascorbic acid (S)
Grams	Grams	Grams	Grams	Grams	Milli- grams	Milli- grams	Milli- grams	Milli- grams	Inter- national units	Milli- grams	Milli- grams	Milli- grams	Milli- grams
Trace	—	—	—	49	36	51	1.8	602	—	.03	.03	1.0	5
Trace	—	—	—	112	90	146	5.1	1,106	30	.16	.12	.7	1
Trace	—	—	—	11	9	14	.5	107	Trace	.02	.01	.1	Trace
1	—	—	—	17	27	27	1.1	207	160	.04	.11	1.1	31
1	—	—	—	70	37	48	1.7	284	200	.06	.17	1.7	60
Trace	—	—	—	97	211	41	1.6	548	220	.05	.14	.8	16
1	—	—	—	98	211	32	1.9	475	190	.05	.11	.5	16
1	—	—	—	13	31	31	1.5	244	90	0.04	0.10	0.9	88
1	—	—	—	79	40	48	2.0	318	90	.06	.17	1.4	151
1	—	—	—	107	59	73	2.7	472	140	.09	.27	2.3	249
Trace	—	—	—	10	34	15	.3	108	360	.05	.02	.1	27
Trace	—	—	—	30	44	35	.5	440	1,040	.15	.05	.2	54
1	—	—	—	27	30	43	2.1	426	2,510	.13	.13	.9	30
2	0.5	0.9	0.8	28	9	43	1.2	41	30	.14	.10	1.2	0
1	.2	.4	.6	30	8	41	1.2	42	0	.15	.11	1.4	0
2	.3	.2	.8	158	32	378	4.0	320	0	.24	.10	6.2	0
5	1.2	2.0	1.2	13	34	49	.4	33	Trace	.08	.08	.7	Trace
3	.6	1.1	.7	15	19	65	.6	32	Trace	.09	.08	.8	Trace
5	1.0	1.6	1.4	73	122	141	3.6	152	Trace	.35	.35	4.8	Trace
1	.1	.2	.2	21	41	72	.9	131	[39]0	.06	.04	.7	0
10	2.2	3.0	3.9	236	399	581	9.5	608	Trace	1.52	1.13	14.4	Trace
1	.1	.2	.2	13	22	32	.5	34	Trace	.08	.06	.8	Trace
14	3.2	4.7	4.6	251	195	386	10.0	408	Trace	1.80	1.10	15.0	Trace
1	.2	.4	.4	19	15	30	.8	32	Trace	.14	.08	1.2	Trace
1	.2	.3	.3	14	11	21	.6	23	Trace	.10	.06	.8	Trace
4	.6	.3	1.5	256	77	349	10.0	336	0	1.80	1.10	15.0	0
Trace	Trace	Trace	.1	17	5	23	.7	22	0	.12	.07	1.0	0

NUTRITIVE VALUES OF THE EDIBLE PART OF FOODS · Continued

(Dashes (—) denote lack of reliable data for a constituent believed to be present in measurable amount)

Item No. (A)	Foods, approximate measures, units, and weight (edible part unless footnotes indicate otherwise) (B)		Water (C)	Food energy (D)	Pro- tein (E)
		Grams	Per- cent	Cal- ories	Grams

GRAIN PRODUCTS —Con.

Breads —Continued
Raisin bread, enriched:[38]

333	Loaf, 1 lb------------------	1 loaf--------------------	454	35	1,190	30
334	Slice (18 per loaf)----------	1 slice--------------------	25	35	65	2
	Rye Bread:					
	American, light (2/3 enriched wheat flour, 1/3 rye flour):					
335	Loaf, 1 lb------------------	1 loaf--------------------	454	36	1,100	41
336	Slice (4 3/4 by 3 3/4 by 7/16 in).	1 slice--------------------	25	36	60	2
	Pumpernickel (2/3 rye flour, 1/3 enriched wheat flour):					
337	Loaf, 1 lb------------------	1 loaf--------------------	454	34	1,115	41
338	Slice (5 by 4 by 3/8 in)----	1 slice--------------------	32	34	80	3
	White bread, enriched:[38]					
	Soft-crumb type:					
339	Loaf, 1 lb------------------	1 loaf--------------------	454	36	1,225	39
340	Slice (18 per loaf)-------	1 slice--------------------	25	36	70	2
341	Slice, toasted----------	1 slice--------------------	22	25	70	2
342	Slice (22 per loaf)-------	1 slice--------------------	20	36	55	2
343	Slice, toasted----------	1 slice--------------------	17	25	55	2
344	Loaf, 1 1/2 lb-------------	1 loaf--------------------	680	36	1,835	59
345	Slice (24 per loaf)-------	1 slice--------------------	28	36	75	2
346	Slice, toasted----------	1 slice--------------------	24	25	75	2
347	Slice (28 per loaf)-------	1 slice--------------------	24	36	65	2
348	Slice, toasted----------	1 slice--------------------	21	25	65	2
349	Cubes-----------------------	1 cup---------------------	30	36	80	3
350	Crumbs----------------------	1 cup---------------------	45	36	120	4
	Firm-crumb type:					
351	Loaf, 1 lb------------------	1 loaf--------------------	454	35	1,245	41
352	Slice (20 per loaf)-------	1 slice--------------------	23	35	65	2
353	Slice, toasted----------	1 slice--------------------	20	24	65	2
354	Loaf, 2 lb------------------	1 loaf--------------------	907	35	2,495	82
355	Slice (34 per loaf)-------	1 slice--------------------	27	35	75	2
356	Slice, toasted----------	1 slice--------------------	23	24	75	2
	Whole-wheat bread:					
	Soft-crumb type:[38]					
357	Loaf, 1 lb------------------	1 loaf--------------------	454	36	1,095	41
358	Slice (16 per loaf)-------	1 slice--------------------	28	36	65	3
359	Slice, toasted----------	1 slice--------------------	24	24	65	3
	Firm-crumb type:[38]					
360	Loaf, 1 lb------------------	1 loaf--------------------	454	36	1,100	48
361	Slice (18 per loaf)-------	1 slice--------------------	25	36	60	3
362	Slice, toasted----------	1 slice--------------------	21	24	60	3
	Breakfast cereals:					
	Hot type, cooked:					
	Corn (hominy) grits, degermed:					
363	Enriched------------------	1 cup---------------------	245	87	125	3
364	Unenriched----------------	1 cup---------------------	245	87	125	3
365	Farina, quick-cooking, en- riched.	1 cup---------------------	245	89	105	3
366	Oatmeal or rolled oats--------	1 cup---------------------	240	87	130	5
367	Wheat, rolled----------------	1 cup---------------------	240	80	180	5
368	Wheat, whole-meal------------	1 cup---------------------	245	88	110	4
	Ready-to-eat:					
369	Bran flakes (40% bran), added sugar, salt, iron, vitamins.	1 cup---------------------	35	3	105	4

[38]Made with vegetable shortening.
[40]Applies to white varieties. For yellow varieties, value is 150 International Units (I.U.).
[41]Applies to products that do not contain di-sodium phosphate. If di-sodium phosphate is an ingredient, value is 162 mg.
[42]Value may range from less than 1 mg to about 8 mg depending on the brand. Consult the label.

		Fatty Acids												
		Unsaturated												
Fat	Satu-rated (total)	Oleic	Lino-leic	Carbo-hydrate	Calcium	Phos-phorus	Iron	Potas-sium	Vitamin A value	Thiamin	Ribo-flavin	Niacin	Ascorbic acid
(F)	(G)	(H)	(I)	(J)	(K)	(L)	(M)	(N)	(O)	(P)	(Q)	(R)	(S)
Grams	Grams	Grams	Grams	Grams	Milli-grams	Milli-grams	Milli-grams	Milli-grams	Inter-national units	Milli-grams	Milli-grams	Milli-grams	Milli-grams
13	3.0	4.7	3.9	243	322	395	10.0	1,057	Trace	1.70	1.07	10.7	Trace
1	.2	.3	.2	13	18	22	.6	58	Trace	.09	.06	.6	Trace
5	0.7	0.5	2.2	236	340	667	9.1	658	0	1.35	0.98	12.9	0
Trace	Trace	Trace	.1	13	19	37	.5	36	0	.07	.05	.7	0
5	.7	.5	2.4	241	381	1,039	11.8	2,059	0	1.30	.93	8.5	0
Trace	.1	Trace	.2	17	27	73	.8	145	0	.09	.07	.6	0
15	3.4	5.3	4.6	229	381	440	11.3	476	Trace	1.80	1.10	15.0	Trace
1	.2	.3	.3	13	21	24	.6	26	Trace	.10	.06	.8	Trace
1	.2	.3	.3	13	21	24	.6	26	Trace	.08	.06	.8	Trace
1	.2	.2	.2	10	17	19	.5	21	Trace	.08	.05	.7	Trace
1	.2	.2	.2	10	17	19	.5	21	Trace	.06	.05	.7	Trace
22	5.2	7.9	6.9	343	571	660	17.0	714	Trace	2.70	1.65	22.5	Trace
1	.2	.3	.3	14	24	27	.7	29	Trace	.11	.07	.9	Trace
1	.2	.3	.3	14	24	27	.7	29	Trace	.09	.07	.9	Trace
1	.2	.3	.2	12	20	23	.6	25	Trace	.10	.06	.8	Trace
1	.2	.3	.2	12	20	23	.6	25	Trace	.08	.06	.8	Trace
1	.2	.3	.3	15	25	29	.8	32	Trace	.12	.07	1.0	Trace
1	.3	.5	.5	23	38	44	1.1	47	Trace	.18	.11	1.5	Trace
17	3.9	5.9	5.2	228	435	463	11.3	549	Trace	1.80	1.10	15.0	Trace
1	.2	.3	.3	12	22	23	.6	28	Trace	.09	.06	.8	Trace
1	.2	.3	.3	12	22	23	.6	28	Trace	.07	.06	.8	Trace
34	7.7	11.8	10.4	455	871	925	22.7	1,097	Trace	3.60	2.20	30.0	Trace
1	.2	.3	.3	14	26	28	.7	33	Trace	.11	.06	.9	Trace
1	.2	.3	.3	14	26	28	.7	33	Trace	.09	.06	.9	Trace
12	2.2	2.9	4.2	224	381	1,152	13.6	1,161	Trace	1.37	.45	12.7	Trace
1	.1	.2	.2	14	24	71	.8	72	Trace	.09	.03	.8	Trace
1	.1	.2	.2	14	24	71	.8	72	Trace	.07	.03	.8	Trace
14	2.5	3.3	4.9	216	449	1,034	13.6	1,238	Trace	1.17	.54	12.7	Trace
1	.1	.2	.3	12	25	57	.8	68	Trace	.06	.03	.7	Trace
1	.1	.2	.3	12	25	57	.8	68	Trace	.05	.03	.7	Trace
Trace	Trace	Trace	.1	27	2	25	.7	27	[40]Trace	.10	.07	1.0	0
Trace	Trace	Trace	.1	27	2	25	.2	27	[40]Trace	.05	.02	.5	0
Trace	Trace	Trace	.1	22	147	[41]113	([42])	25	0	.12	.07	1.0	0
2	.4	.8	.9	23	22	137	1.4	146	0	.19	.05	.2	0
1	—	—	—	41	19	182	1.7	202	0	.17	.07	2.2	0
1	—	—	—	23	17	127	1.2	118	0	.15	.05	1.5	0
1	—	—	—	28	19	125	5.6	137	1,540	.46	.52	6.2	0

NUTRITIVE VALUES OF THE EDIBLE PART OF FOODS · Continued

(Dashes (—) denote lack of reliable data for a constituent believed to be present in measurable amount)

Item No. (A)	Foods, approximate measures, units, and weight (edible part unless footnotes indicate otherwise) (B)		Water (C)	Food energy (D)	Pro-tein (E)
		Grams	Per-cent	Cal-ories	Grams

GRAIN PRODUCTS—Con.

Breakfast cereals—Continued
Ready-to-eat—Continued

370	Bran flakes with raisins, add- ed sugar, salt, iron, vita- mins.	1 cup----------------------	50	7	145	4
	Corn flakes:					
371	Plain, added sugar, salt, iron, vitamins.	1 cup----------------------	25	4	95	2
372	Sugar-coated, added salt, iron, vitamins.	1 cup----------------------	40	2	155	2
373	Corn, oat flour, puffed, added sugar, salt, iron, vita- mins.	1 cup----------------------	20	4	80	2
374	Corn, shredded, added sugar, salt, iron, thiamin, niacin.	1 cup----------------------	25	3	95	2
375	Oats, puffed, added sugar, salt, minerals, vitamins.	1 cup----------------------	25	3	100	3
	Rice, puffed:					
376	Plain, added iron, thiamin, niacin.	1 cup----------------------	15	4	60	1
377	Presweetened, added salt, iron, vitamins.	1 cup----------------------	28	3	115	1
378	Wheat flakes, added sugar, salt, iron, vitamins.	1 cup----------------------	30	4	105	3
	Wheat, puffed:					
379	Plain, added iron, thiamin, niacin.	1 cup----------------------	15	3	55	2
380	Presweetened, added salt, iron, vitamins.	1 cup----------------------	38	3	140	3
381	Wheat, shredded, plain-------	1 oblong biscuit or 1/2 cup spoon-size biscuits.	25	7	90	2
382	Wheat germ, without salt and sugar, toasted.	1 tbsp--------------------	6	4	25	2
383	Buckwheat flour, light, sifted-	1 cup----------------------	98	12	340	6
384	Bulgur, canned, seasoned----------	1 cup----------------------	135	56	245	8
	Cake icings. See Sugars and Sweets (items 532-536). Cakes made from cake mixes with enriched flour:[46] Angelfood:					
385	Whole cake (9 3/4-in diam. tube cake).	1 cake---------------------	635	34	1,645	36
386	Piece, 1/12 of cake----------	1 piece--------------------	53	34	135	3
	Coffeecake:					
387	Whole cake (7 3/4 by 5 5/8 by 1 1/4 in).	1 cake---------------------	430	30	1,385	27
388	Piece, 1/6 of cake-----------	1 piece--------------------	72	30	230	5
	Cupcakes, made with egg, milk, 2 1/2-in diam.:					
389	Without icing---------------	1 cupcake-----------------	25	26	90	1
390	With chocolate icing--------	1 cupcake-----------------	36	22	130	2
	Devil's food with chocolate icing:					
391	Whole, 2 layer cake (8- or 9-in diam.).	1 cake---------------------	1,107	24	3,755	49
392	Piece, 1/16 of cake----------	1 piece--------------------	69	24	235	3
393	Cupcake, 2 1/2-in diam-------	1 cupcake-----------------	35	24	120	2

[43] Applies to product with added nutrient. Without added nutrient, value is trace.
[44] Value varies with the brand. Consult the label.
[45] Applies to product with added nutrient. Without added nutrient, value is trace.
[46] Excepting angelfood cake, cakes were made from mixes containing vegetable shortening; icings, with butter.

		Fatty Acids											
Fat	Satu-rated (total)	Unsaturated Oleic	Unsaturated Lino-leic	Carbo-hydrate	Calcium	Phos-phorus	Iron	Potas-sium	Vitamin A value	Thiamin	Ribo-flavin	Niacin	Ascorbic acid
(F)	(G)	(H)	(I)	(J)	(K)	(L)	(M)	(N)	(O)	(P)	(Q)	(R)	(S)
Grams	Grams	Grams	Grams	Grams	Milli-grams	Milli-grams	Milli-grams	Milli-grams	Inter-national units	Milli-grams	Milli-grams	Milli-grams	Milli-grams
1	—	—	—	40	28	146	7.9	154	[45]2,200	([44])	([44])	([44])	0
Trace	—	—	—	21	([44])	9	([44])	30	([44])	([44])	([44])	([44])	[45]13
Trace	—	—	—	37	1	10	([44])	27	1,760	.53	.60	7.1	[45]21
1	—	—	—	16	4	18	5.7	—	880	.26	.30	3.5	11
Trace	—	—	—	22	1	10	.6	—	0	.33	.05	4.4	13
1	—	—	—	19	44	102	4.0	—	1,100	.33	.38	4.4	13
Trace	—	—	—	13	3	14	.3	15	0	.07	.01	.7	0
0	—	—	—	26	3	14	([44])	43	[45]1,240	([44])	([44])	([44])	[45]15
Trace	—	—	—	24	12	83	4.8	81	1,320	.40	.45	5.3	16
Trace	—	—	—	12	4	48	.6	51	0	.08	.03	1.2	0
Trace	—	—	—	33	7	52	([44])	63	1,680	.50	.57	6.7	[45]20
1	—	—	—	20	11	97	.9	87	0	.06	.03	1.1	0
1	—	—	—	3	3	70	.5	57	10	.11	.05	.3	1
1	0.2	0.4	0.4	78	11	86	1.0	314	0	.08	.04	.4	0
4	—	—	—	44	27	263	1.9	151	0	.08	.05	4.1	0
1	—	—	—	377	603	756	2.5	381	0	.37	.95	3.6	0
Trace	—	—	—	32	50	63	.2	32	0	.03	.08	.3	0
41	11.7	16.3	8.8	225	262	748	6.9	469	690	.82	.91	7.7	1
7	2.0	2.7	1.5	38	44	125	1.2	78	120	.14	.15	1.3	Trace
3	.8	1.2	.7	14	40	59	.3	21	40	.05	.05	.4	Trace
5	2.0	1.6	.6	21	47	71	.4	42	60	.05	.06	.4	Trace
136	50.0	44.9	17.0	645	653	1,162	16.6	1,439	1,660	1.06	1.65	10.1	1
8	3.1	2.8	1.1	40	41	72	1.0	90	100	.07	.10	.6	Trace
4	1.6	1.4	.5	20	21	37	.5	46	50	.03	.05	.3	Trace

NUTRITIVE VALUES OF THE EDIBLE PART OF FOODS · Continued

(Dashes (—) denote lack of reliable data for a constituent believed to be present in measurable amount)

Item No. (A)	Foods, approximate measures, units, and weight (edible part unless footnotes indicate otherwise) (B)		Water (C)	Food energy (D)	Pro-tein (E)
		Grams	Per-cent	Cal-ories	Grams
	GRAIN PRODUCTS—Con.				
	Cakes made from cake mixes with enriched flour:[46]—Continued				
	Gingerbread:				
394	Whole cake (8-in square)------- 1 cake--------------------	570	37	1,575	18
395	Piece, 1/9 of cake------------- 1 piece-------------------	63	37	175	2
	White, 2 layer with chocolate icing:				
396	Whole cake (8- or 9-in diam.)-- 1 cake--------------------	1,140	21	4,000	44
397	Piece, 1/16 of cake------------ 1 piece-------------------	71	21	250	3
	Yellow, 2 layer with chocolate icing:				
398	Whole cake (8- or 9-in diam.)-- 1 cake--------------------	1,108	26	3,735	45
399	Piece, 1/16 of cake------------ 1 piece-------------------	69	26	235	3
	Cakes made from home recipes using enriched flour:[47]				
	Boston cream pie with custard filling:				
400	Whole cake (8-in diam.)-------- 1 cake--------------------	825	35	2,490	41
401	Piece, 1/12 of cake------------ 1 piece-------------------	69	35	210	3
	Fruitcake, dark:				
402	Loaf, 1-lb (7 1/2 by 2 by 1 1/2 in). 1 loaf--------------------	454	18	1,720	22
403	Slice, 1/30 of loaf------------ 1 slice------------------	15	18	55	1
	Plain, sheet cake:				
	Without icing:				
404	Whole cake (9-in square)------ 1 cake--------------------	777	25	2,830	35
405	Piece, 1/9 of cake------------- 1 piece-------------------	86	25	315	4
	With uncooked white icing:				
406	Whole cake (9-in square)------ 1 cake--------------------	1,096	21	4,020	37
407	Piece, 1/9 of cake------------- 1 piece-------------------	121	21	445	4
408	Pound:[49] Loaf, 8 1/2 by 3 1/2 by 3 1/4 in. 1 loaf--------------------	565	16	2,725	31
409	Slice, 1/17 of loaf------------ 1 slice------------------	33	16	160	2
	Spongecake:				
410	Whole cake (9 3/4-in diam. tube cake). 1 cake--------------------	790	32	2,345	60
411	Piece, 1/12 of cake------------ 1 piece-------------------	66	32	195	5
	Cookies made with enriched flour:[50][51]				
	Brownies with nuts:				
	Home-prepared, 1 3/4 by 1 3/4 by 7/8 in:				
412	From home recipe------------- 1 brownie----------------	20	10	95	1
413	From commercial recipe------- 1 brownie----------------	20	11	85	1
414	Frozen, with chocolate icing,[52] 1 brownie---------------- 1 1/2 by 1 3/4 by 7/8 in.	25	13	105	1
	Chocolate chip:				
415	Commercial, 2 1/4-in diam., 3/8 4 cookies---------------- in thick.	42	3	200	2
416	From home recipe, 2 1/3-in diam. 4 cookies----------------	40	3	205	2
417	Fig bars, square (1 5/8 by 1 5/8 4 cookies---------------- by 3/8 in) or rectangular (1 1/2 by 1 3/4 by 1/2 in).	56	14	200	2
418	Gingersnaps, 2-in diam., 1/4 in 4 cookies---------------- thick.	28	3	90	2

[46]Excepting angelfood cake, cakes were made from mixes containing vegetable shortening; icings, with butter.

[47]Excepting spongecake, vegetable shortening used for cake portion; butter, for icing. If butter or margarine used for cake portion, vitamin A values would be higher.

[48]Applies to product made with a sodium aluminum-sulfate type baking powder. With a low-sodium type baking powder containing potassium, value would be about twice the amount shown.

[49]Equal weights of flour, sugar, eggs, and vegetable shortening.

[50]Products are commercial unless otherwise specified.

[51]Made with enriched flour and vegetable shortening except for macaroons which do not contain flour or shortening.

[52]Icing made with butter.

		NUTRIENTS IN INDICATED QUANTITY											
Fat	Satu-rated (total)	Fatty Acids		Carbo-hydrate	Calcium	Phos-phorus	Iron	Potas-sium	Vitamin A value	Thiamin	Ribo-flavin	Niacin	Ascorbic acid
		Unsaturated											
		Oleic	Lino-leic										
(F)	(G)	(H)	(I)	(J)	(K)	(L)	(M)	(N)	(O)	(P)	(Q)	(R)	(S)
Grams	Grams	Grams	Grams	Grams	Milli-grams	Milli-grams	Milli-grams	Milli-grams	Inter-national units	Milli-grams	Milli-grams	Milli-grams	Milli-grams
39	9.7	16.6	10.0	291	513	570	8.6	1,562	Trace	0.84	1.00	7.4	Trace
4	1.1	1.8	1.1	32	57	63	.9	173	Trace	.09	.11	.8	Trace
122	48.2	46.4	20.0	716	1,129	2,041	11.4	1,322	680	1.50	1.77	12.5	2
8	3.0	2.9	1.2	45	70	127	.7	82	40	.09	.11	.8	Trace
125	47.8	47.8	20.3	638	1,008	2,017	12.2	1,208	1,550	1.24	1.67	10.6	2
8	3.0	3.0	1.3	40	63	126	.8	75	100	.08	.10	.7	Trace
78	23.0	30.1	15.2	412	553	833	8.2	[48]734	1,730	1.04	1.27	9.6	2
6	1.9	2.5	1.3	34	46	70	.7	[48]61	140	.09	.11	.8	Trace
69	14.4	33.5	14.8	271	327	513	11.8	2,250	540	.72	.73	4.9	2
2	.5	1.1	.5	9	11	17	.4	74	20	.02	.02	.2	Trace
108	29.5	44.4	23.9	434	497	793	8.5	[48]614	1,320	1.21	1.40	10.2	2
12	3.3	4.9	2.6	48	55	88	.9	[48]68	150	.13	.15	1.1	Trace
129	42.2	49.5	24.4	694	548	822	8.2	[48]669	2,190	1.22	1.47	10.2	2
14	4.7	5.5	2.7	77	61	91	.8	[48]74	240	.14	.16	1.1	Trace
170	42.9	73.1	39.6	273	107	418	7.9	345	1,410	.90	.99	7.3	0
10	2.5	4.3	2.3	16	6	24	.5	20	80	.05	.06	.4	0
45	13.1	15.8	5.7	427	237	885	13.4	687	3,560	1.10	1.64	7.4	Trace
4	1.1	1.3	.5	36	20	74	1.1	57	300	.09	.14	.6	Trace
6	1.5	3.0	1.2	10	8	30	.4	38	40	.04	.03	.2	Trace
4	.9	1.4	1.3	13	9	27	.4	34	20	.03	.02	.2	Trace
5	2.0	2.2	.7	15	10	31	.4	44	50	.03	.03	.2	Trace
9	2.8	2.9	2.2	29	16	48	1.0	56	50	.10	.17	.9	Trace
12	3.5	4.5	2.9	24	14	40	.8	47	40	.06	.06	.5	Trace
3	.8	1.2	.7	42	44	34	1.0	111	60	.04	.14	.9	Trace
2	.7	1.0	.6	22	20	13	.7	129	20	.08	.06	.7	0

NUTRITIVE VALUES OF THE EDIBLE PART OF FOODS · Continued

(Dashes (—) denote lack of reliable data for a constituent believed to be present in measurable amount)

Item No. (A)	Foods, approximate measures, units, and weight (edible part unless footnotes indicate otherwise) (B)		Water (C)	Food energy (D)	Pro- tein (E)
		Grams	Per- cent	Cal- ories	Grams

GRAIN PRODUCTS—Con.

	Cookies made with enriched flour[50][51]—Continued				
419	Macaroons, 2 3/4-in diam., 1/4 in thick.	2 cookies----------------	38	4	180	2
420	Oatmeal with raisins, 2 5/8-in diam., 1/4 in thick.	4 cookies----------------	52	3	235	3
421	Plain, prepared from commercial chilled dough, 2 1/2-in diam., 1/4 in thick.	4 cookies----------------	48	5	240	2
422	Sandwich type (chocolate or vanilla), 1 3/4-in diam., 3/8 in thick.	4 cookies----------------	40	2	200	2
423	Vanilla wafers, 1 3/4-in diam., 1/4 in thick.	10 cookies---------------	40	3	185	2
	Cornmeal:					
424	Whole-ground, unbolted, dry form.	1 cup--------------------	122	12	435	11
425	Bolted (nearly whole-grain), dry form.	1 cup--------------------	122	12	440	11
	Degermed, enriched:					
426	Dry form----------------------	1 cup--------------------	138	12	500	11
427	Cooked------------------------	1 cup--------------------	240	88	120	3
	Degermed, unenriched:					
428	Dry form----------------------	1 cup--------------------	138	12	500	11
429	Cooked------------------------	1 cup--------------------	240	88	120	3
	Crackers:[38]					
430	Graham, plain, 2 1/2-in square--	2 crackers---------------	14	6	55	1
431	Rye wafers, whole-grain, 1 7/8 by 3 1/2 in.	2 wafers-----------------	13	6	45	2
432	Saltines, made with enriched flour.	4 crackers or 1 packet---	11	4	50	1
	Danish pastry (enriched flour), plain without fruit or nuts:[54]					
433	Packaged ring, 12 oz------------	1 ring-------------------	340	22	1,435	25
434	Round piece, about 4 1/4-in diam. by 1 in.	1 pastry-----------------	65	22	275	5
435	Ounce--------------------------	1 oz---------------------	28	22	120	2
	Doughnuts, made with enriched flour:[38]					
436	Cake type, plain, 2 1/2-in diam., 1 in high.	1 doughnut---------------	25	24	100	1
437	Yeast-leavened, glazed, 3 3/4-in diam., 1 1/4 in high.	1 doughnut---------------	50	26	205	3
	Macaroni, enriched, cooked (cut lengths, elbows, shells):					
438	Firm stage (hot)---------------	1 cup--------------------	130	64	190	7
	Tender stage:					
439	Cold macaroni-----------------	1 cup--------------------	105	73	115	4
440	Hot macaroni------------------	1 cup--------------------	140	73	155	5
	Macaroni (enriched) and cheese:					
441	Canned[55]----------------------	1 cup--------------------	240	80	230	9
442	From home recipe (served hot)[56]-	1 cup--------------------	200	58	430	17
	Muffins made with enriched flour:[38]					
	From home recipe:					
443	Blueberry, 2 3/8-in diam., 1 1/2 in high.	1 muffin-----------------	40	39	110	3

[38]Made with vegetable shortening.
[50]Products are commercial unless otherwise specified.
[51]Made with enriched flour and vegetable shortening except for macaroons which do not contain flour or shortening.
[53]Applies to yellow varieties; white varieties contain only a trace.
[54]Contains vegetable shortening and butter.
[55]Made with corn oil.
[56]Made with regular margarine.

Fat	Fatty Acids			Carbo-hydrate	Calcium	Phos-phorus	Iron	Potas-sium	Vitamin A value	Thiamin	Ribo-flavin	Niacin	Ascorbic acid
	Satu-rated (total)	Unsaturated											
		Oleic	Lino-leic										
(F)	(G)	(H)	(I)	(J)	(K)	(L)	(M)	(N)	(O)	(P)	(Q)	(R)	(S)
Grams	Grams	Grams	Grams	Grams	Milli-grams	Milli-grams	Milli-grams	Milli-grams	Inter-national units	Milli-grams	Milli-grams	Milli-grams	Milli-grams
9	—	—	—	25	10	32	.3	176	0	.02	.06	.2	0
8	2.0	3.3	2.0	38	11	53	1.4	192	30	.15	.10	1.0	Trace
12	3.0	5.2	2.9	31	17	35	0.6	23	30	0.10	0.08	0.9	0
9	2.2	3.9	2.2	28	10	96	.7	15	0	.06	.10	.7	0
6	—	—	—	30	16	25	.6	29	50	.10	.09	.8	0
5	.5	1.0	2.5	90	24	312	2.9	346	[53]620	.46	.13	2.4	0
4	.5	.9	2.1	91	21	272	2.2	303	[53]590	.37	.10	2.3	0
2	.2	.4	.9	108	8	137	4.0	166	[53]610	.61	.36	4.8	0
Trace	Trace	.1	.2	26	2	34	1.0	38	[53]140	.14	.10	1.2	0
2	.2	.4	.9	108	8	137	1.5	166	[53]610	.19	.07	1.4	0
Trace	Trace	.1	.2	26	2	34	.5	38	[53]140	.05	.02	.2	0
1	.3	.5	.3	10	6	21	.5	55	0	.02	.08	.5	0
Trace	—	—	—	10	7	50	.5	78	0	.04	.03	.2	0
1	.3	.5	.4	8	2	10	.5	13	0	.05	.05	.4	0
80	24.3	31.7	16.5	155	170	371	6.1	381	1,050	.97	1.01	8.6	Trace
15	4.7	6.1	3.2	30	33	71	1.2	73	200	.18	.19	1.7	Trace
7	2.0	2.7	1.4	13	14	31	.5	32	90	.08	.08	.7	Trace
5	1.2	2.0	1.1	13	10	48	.4	23	20	.05	.05	.4	Trace
11	3.3	5.8	3.3	22	16	33	.6	34	25	.10	.10	.8	0
1	—	—	—	39	14	85	1.4	103	0	.23	.13	1.8	0
Trace	—	—	—	24	8	53	.9	64	0	.15	.08	1.2	0
1	—	—	—	32	11	70	1.3	85	.0	.20	.11	1.5	0
10	4.2	3.1	1.4	26	199	182	1.0	139	260	.12	.24	1.0	Trace
22	8.9	8.8	2.9	40	362	322	1.8	240	860	.20	.40	1.8	Trace
4	1.1	1.4	.7	17	34	53	.6	46	90	.09	.10	.7	Trace

NUTRITIVE VALUES OF THE EDIBLE PART OF FOODS - Continued

(Dashes (—) denote lack of reliable data for a constituent believed to be present in measurable amount)

Item No. (A)	Foods, approximate measures, units, and weight (edible part unless footnotes indicate otherwise) (B)		Water (C)	Food energy (D)	Pro- tein (E)
		Grams	Per- cent	Cal- ories	Grams

GRAIN PRODUCTS—Con.

	Muffins made with enriched flour:[38] —Continued				
	From home recipe —Continued				
444	Bran------------------------- 1 muffin-------------------	40	35	105	3
445	Corn (enriched degermed corn-meal and flour), 2 3/8-in diam., 1 1/2 in high. 1 muffin-------------------	40	33	125	3
446	Plain, 3-in diam., 1 1/2 in high. 1 muffin-------------------	40	38	120	3
	From mix, egg, milk:				
447	Corn, 2 3/8-in diam., 1 1/2 in high.[58] 1 muffin-------------------	40	30	130	3
448	Noodles (egg noodles), enriched, cooked. 1 cup------------------------	160	71	200	7
449	Noodles, chow mein, canned--------- 1 cup---------------------	45	1	220	6
	Pancakes, (4-in diam.):[38]				
450	Buckwheat, made from mix (with buckwheat and enriched flours), egg and milk added. 1 cake--------------------	27	58	55	2
	Plain:				
•51	Made from home recipe using enriched flour. 1 cake--------------------	27	50	60	2
452	Made from mix with enriched flour, egg and milk added. 1 cake--------------------	27	51	60	2
	Pies, piecrust made with enriched flour, vegetable shortening (9-in diam.):				
	Apple:				
453	Whole--------------------------- 1 pie---------------------	945	48	2,420	21
454	Sector, 1/7 of pie------------- 1 sector-------------------	135	48	345	3
	Banana cream:				
455	Whole--------------------------- 1 pie---------------------	910	54	2,010	41
456	Sector, 1/7 of pie-------------- 1 sector-------------------	130	54	285	6
	Blueberry:				
457	Whole--------------------------- 1 pie---------------------	945	51	2,285	23
458	Sector, 1/7 of pie------------- 1 sector-------------------	135	51	325	3
	Cherry:				
459	Whole--------------------------- 1 pie---------------------	945	47	2,465	25
460	Sector, 1/7 of pie------------- 1 sector-------------------	135	47	350	4
	Custard:				
461	Whole--------------------------- 1 pie---------------------	910	58	1,985	56
462	Sector, 1/7 of pie------------- 1 sector-------------------	130	58	285	8
	Lemon meringue:				
463	Whole--------------------------- 1 pie---------------------	840	47	2,140	31
464	Sector, 1/7 of pie------------- 1 sector-------------------	120	47	305	4
	Mince:				
465	Whole--------------------------- 1 pie---------------------	945	43	2,560	24
466	Sector, 1/7 of pie------------- 1 sector-------------------	135	43	365	3
	Peach:				
467	Whole--------------------------- 1 pie---------------------	945	48	2,410	24
468	Sector, 1/7 of pie------------- 1 sector-------------------	135	48	345	3
	Pecan:				
469	Whole--------------------------- 1 pie---------------------	825	20	3,450	42
470	Sector, 1/7 of pie------------- 1 sector-------------------	118	20	495	6
	Pumpkin:				
471	Whole--------------------------- 1 pie---------------------	910	59	1,920	36
472	Sector, 1/7 of pie------------- 1 sector-------------------	130	59	275	5
473	Piecrust (home recipe) made with enriched flour and vegetable shortening, baked. 1 pie shell, 9-in diam.---	180	15	900	11

[38]Made with vegetable shortening.
[57]Applies to product made with yellow cornmeal.
[58]Made with enriched degermed cornmeal and enriched flour.

		NUTRIENTS IN INDICATED QUANTITY											
	Fatty Acids												
Fat	Saturated (total)	Unsaturated		Carbohydrate	Calcium	Phosphorus	Iron	Potassium	Vitamin A value	Thiamin	Riboflavin	Niacin	Ascorbic acid
		Oleic	Linoleic										
(F)	(G)	(H)	(I)	(J)	(K)	(L)	(M)	(N)	(O)	(P)	(Q)	(R)	(S)
Grams	Grams	Grams	Grams	Grams	Milligrams	Milligrams	Milligrams	Milligrams	International units	Milligrams	Milligrams	Milligrams	Milligrams
4	1.2	1.4	.8	17	57	162	1.5	172	90	.07	.10	1.7	Trace
4	1.2	1.6	.9	19	42	68	.7	54	[57]120	.10	.10	.7	Trace
4	1.0	1.7	1.0	17	42	60	0.6	50	40	0.09	0.12	0.9	Trace
4	1.2	1.7	.9	20	96	152	.6	44	[57]100	.08	.09	.7	Trace
2	—	—	—	37	16	94	1.4	70	110	.22	.13	1.9	0
11	—	—	—	26	—	—	—	—	—	—	—	—	—
2	.8	.9	.4	6	59	91	.4	66	60	.04	.05	.2	Trace
2	.5	.8	.5	9	27	38	.4	33	30	.06	.07	.5	Trace
2	.7	.7	.3	9	58	70	.3	42	70	.04	.06	.2	Trace
105	27.0	44.5	25.2	360	76	208	6.6	756	280	1.06	.79	9.3	9
15	3.9	6.4	3.6	51	11	30	.9	108	40	.15	.11	1.3	2
85	26.7	33.2	16.2	279	601	746	7.3	1,847	2,280	.77	1.51	7.0	9
12	3.8	4.7	2.3	40	86	107	1.0	264	330	.11	.22	1.0	1
102	24.8	43.7	25.1	330	104	217	9.5	614	280	1.03	.80	10.0	28
15	3.5	6.2	3.6	47	31	31	1.4	88	40	.15	.11	1.4	4
107	28.2	45.0	25.3	363	132	236	6.6	992	4,160	1.09	.84	9.8	Trace
15	4.0	6.4	3.6	52	19	34	.9	142	590	.16	.12	1.4	Trace
101	33.9	38.5	17.5	213	874	1,028	8.2	1,247	2,090	.79	1.92	5.6	0
14	4.8	5.5	2.5	30	125	147	1.2	178	300	.11	.27	.8	0
86	26.1	33.8	16.4	317	118	412	6.7	420	1,430	.61	.84	5.2	25
12	3.7	4.8	2.3	45	17	59	1.0	60	200	.09	.12	.7	4
109	28.0	45.9	25.2	389	265	359	13.3	1,682	20	.96	.86	9.8	9
16	4.0	6.6	3.6	56	38	51	1.9	240	Trace	.14	.12	1.4	1
101	24.8	43.7	25.1	361	95	274	8.5	1,408	6,900	1.04	.97	14.0	28
14	3.5	6.2	3.6	52	14	39	1.2	201	990	.15	.14	2.0	4
189	27.8	101.0	44.2	423	388	850	25.6	1,015	1,320	1.80	.95	6.9	Trace
27	4.0	14.4	6.3	61	55	122	3.7	145	190	.26	.14	1.0	Trace
102	37.4	37.5	16.6	223	464	628	7.3	1,456	22,480	.78	1.27	7.0	Trace
15	5.4	5.4	2.4	32	66	90	1.0	208	3,210	.11	.18	1.0	Trace
60	14.8	26.1	14.9	79	25	90	3.1	89	0	.47	.40	5.0	0

NUTRITIVE VALUES OF THE EDIBLE PART OF FOODS · Continued

(Dashes (—) denote lack of reliable data for a constituent believed to be present in measurable amount)

Item No. (A)	Foods, approximate measures, units, and weight (edible part unless footnotes indicate otherwise) (B)		Water (C)	Food energy (D)	Pro-tein (E)
		Grams	Per-cent	Cal-ories	Grams

GRAIN PRODUCTS—Con.

474	Piecrust mix with enriched flour and vegetable shortening, 10-oz pkg. prepared and baked.	Piecrust for 2-crust pie, 9-in diam.	320	19	1,485	20
475	Pizza (cheese) baked, 4 3/4-in sector; 1/8 of 12-in diam. pie.[19]	1 sector-----------------	60	45	145	6
	Popcorn, popped:					
476	Plain, large kernel------------	1 cup--------------------	6	4	25	1
477	With oil (coconut) and salt added, large kernel.	1 cup--------------------	9	3	40	1
478	Sugar coated-------------------	1 cup--------------------	35	4	135	2
	Pretzels, made with enriched flour:					
479	Dutch, twisted, 2 3/4 by 2 5/8 in.	1 pretzel----------------	16	5	60	2
480	Thin, twisted, 3 1/4 by 2 1/4 by 1/4 in.	10 pretzels--------------	60	5	235	6
481	Stick, 2 1/4 in long-----------	10 pretzels--------------	3	5	10	Trace
	Rice, white, enriched:					
482	Instant, ready-to-serve, hot---	1 cup--------------------	165	73	180	4
	Long grain:					
483	Raw---------------------------	1 cup--------------------	185	12	670	12
484	Cooked, served hot-----------	1 cup--------------------	205	73	225	4
	Parboiled:					
485	Raw---------------------------	1 cup--------------------	185	10	685	14
486	Cooked, served hot-----------	1 cup--------------------	175	73	185	4
	Rolls, enriched:[38]					
	Commercial:					
487	Brown-and-serve (12 per 12-oz pkg.), browned.	1 roll--------------------	26	27	85	2
488	Cloverleaf or pan, 2 1/2-in diam., 2 in high.	1 roll--------------------	28	31	85	2
489	Frankfurter and hamburger (8 per 11 1/2-oz pkg.).	1 roll--------------------	40	31	120	3
490	Hard, 3 3/4-in diam., 2 in high.	1 roll--------------------	50	25	155	5
491	Hoagie or submarine, 11 1/2 by 3 by 2 1/2 in.	1 roll--------------------	135	31	390	12
	From home recipe:					
492	Cloverleaf, 2 1/2-in diam., 2 in high.	1 roll--------------------	35	26	120	3
	Spaghetti, enriched, cooked:					
493	Firm stage, "al dente," served hot.	1 cup--------------------	130	64	190	7
494	Tender stage, served hot-------	1 cup--------------------	140	73	155	5
	Spaghetti (enriched) in tomato sauce with cheese:					
495	From home recipe---------------	1 cup--------------------	250	77	260	9
496	Canned-------------------------	1 cup--------------------	250	80	190	6
	Spaghetti (enriched) with meat balls and tomato sauce:					
497	From home recipe---------------	1 cup--------------------	248	70	330	19
498	Canned-------------------------	1 cup--------------------	250	78	260	12
499	Toaster pastries----------------	1 pastry-----------------	50	12	200	3
	Waffles, made with enriched flour, 7-in diam.:[38]					
500	From home recipe---------------	1 waffle-----------------	75	41	210	7
501	From mix, egg and milk added---	1 waffle-----------------	75	42	205	7

[19] Crust made with vegetable shortening and enriched flour.
[38] Made with vegetable shortening.
[59] Product may or may not be enriched with riboflavin. Consult the label.
[60] Value varies with the brand. Consult the label.

Fat	Satu-rated (total)	Unsaturated Oleic	Lino-leic	Carbo-hydrate	Calcium	Phos-phorus	Iron	Potas-sium	Vitamin A value	Thiamin	Ribo-flavin	Niacin	Ascorbic acid
(F)	(G)	(H)	(I)	(J)	(K)	(L)	(M)	(N)	(O)	(P)	(Q)	(R)	(S)
Grams	Grams	Grams	Grams	Grams	Milli-grams	Milli-grams	Milli-grams	Milli-grams	Inter-national units	Milli-grams	Milli-grams	Milli-grams	Milli-grams
93	22.7	39.7	23.4	141	131	272	6.1	179	0	1.07	.79	9.9	0
4	1.7	1.5	0.6	22	86	89	1.1	67	230	0.16	0.18	1.6	4
Trace	Trace	.1	.2	5	1	17	.2	—	—	—	.01	.1	0
2	1.5	.2	.2	5	1	19	.2	—	—	—	.01	.2	0
1	.5	.2	.4	30	2	47	.5	—	—	—	.02	.4	0
1	—	—	—	12	4	21	.2	21	0	.05	.04	.7	0
3	—	—	—	46	13	79	.9	78	0	.20	.15	2.5	0
Trace	—	—	—	2	1	4	Trace	4	0	.01	.01	.1	0
Trace	Trace	Trace	Trace	40	5	31	1.3	—	0	.21	(59)	1.7	0
1	.2	.2	.2	149	44	174	5.4	170	0	.81	.06	6.5	0
Trace	.1	.1	.1	50	21	57	1.8	57	0	.23	.02	2.1	0
1	.2	.1	.2	150	111	370	5.4	278	0	.81	.07	6.5	0
Trace	.1	.1	.1	41	33	100	1.4	75	0	.19	.02	2.1	0
2	.4	.7	.5	14	20	23	.5	25	Trace	.10	.06	.9	Trace
2	.4	.6	.4	15	21	24	.5	27	Trace	.11	.07	.9	Trace
2	.5	.8	.6	21	30	34	.8	38	Trace	.16	.10	1.3	Trace
2	.4	.6	.5	30	24	46	1.2	49	Trace	.20	.12	1.7	Trace
4	.9	1.4	1.4	75	58	115	3.0	122	Trace	.54	.32	4.5	Trace
3	.8	1.1	.7	20	16	36	.7	41	30	.12	.12	1.2	Trace
1	—	—	—	39	14	85	1.4	103	0	.23	.13	1.8	0
1	—	—	—	32	11	70	1.3	85	0	.20	.11	1.5	0
9	2.0	5.4	.7	37	80	135	2.3	408	1,080	.25	.18	2.3	13
2	.5	.3	.4	39	40	88	2.8	303	930	.35	.28	4.5	10
12	3.3	6.3	.9	39	124	236	3.7	665	1,590	.25	.30	4.0	22
10	2.2	3.3	3.9	29	53	113	3.3	245	1,000	.15	.18	2.3	5
6	—	—	—	36	[60]54	[60]67	1.9	[60]74	500	.16	.17	2.1	(60)
7	2.3	2.8	1.4	28	85	130	1.3	109	250	.17	.23	1.4	Trace
8	2.8	2.9	1.2	27	179	257	1.0	146	170	.14	.22	.9	Trace

NUTRITIVE VALUES OF THE EDIBLE PART OF FOODS · Continued

(Dashes (—) denote lack of reliable data for a constituent believed to be present in measurable amount)

Item No. (A)	Foods, approximate measures, units, and weight (edible part unless footnotes indicate otherwise) (B)		Water (C)	Food energy (D)	Pro-tein (E)
		Grams	Per-cent	Cal-ories	Grams
	GRAIN PRODUCTS—Con.				
	Wheat flours:				
	All-purpose or family flour, enriched:				
502	Sifted, spooned--------------- 1 cup--------------------	115	12	420	12
503	Unsifted, spooned------------- 1 cup--------------------	125	12	455	13
504	Cake or pastry flour, enriched, 1 cup-------------------- sifted, spooned.	96	12	350	7
505	Self-rising, enriched, unsifted, 1 cup-------------------- spooned.	125	12	440	12
506	Whole-wheat, from hard wheats, 1 cup-------------------- stirred.	120	12	400	16
	LEGUMES (DRY), NUTS, SEEDS; RELATED PRODUCTS				
	Almonds, shelled:				
507	Chopped (about 130 almonds)----- 1 cup--------------------	130	5	775	24
508	Slivered, not pressed down 1 cup-------------------- (about 115 almonds).	115	5	690	21
	Beans, dry:				
	Common varieties as Great North-ern, navy, and others:				
	Cooked, drained:				
509	Great Northern------------- 1 cup--------------------	180	69	210	14
510	Pea (navy)----------------- 1 cup--------------------	190	69	225	15
	Canned, solids and liquid:				
	White with—				
511	Frankfurters (sliced)----- 1 cup--------------------	255	71	365	19
512	Pork and tomato sauce----- 1 cup--------------------	255	71	310	16
513	Pork and sweet sauce------ 1 cup--------------------	255	66	385	16
514	Red kidney---------------- 1 cup--------------------	255	76	230	15
515	Lima, cooked, drained----------- 1 cup--------------------	190	64	260	16
516	Blackeye peas, dry, cooked (with 1 cup-------------------- residual cooking liquid).	250	80	190	13
517	Brazil nuts, shelled (6-8 large 1 oz--------------------- kernels).	28	5	185	4
518	Cashew nuts, roasted in oil------- 1 cup--------------------	140	5	785	24
	Coconut meat, fresh:				
519	Piece, about 2 by 2 by 1/2 in--- 1 piece-------------------	45	51	155	2
520	Shredded or grated, not pressed 1 cup-------------------- down.	80	51	275	3
521	Filberts (hazelnuts), chopped 1 cup-------------------- (about 80 kernels).	115	6	730	14
522	Lentils, whole, cooked------------ 1 cup--------------------	200	72	210	16
523	Peanuts, roasted in oil, salted 1 cup-------------------- (whole, halves, chopped).	144	2	840	37
524	Peanut butter--------------------- 1 tbsp-------------------	16	2	95	4
525	Peas, split, dry, cooked---------- 1 cup--------------------	200	70	230	16
526	Pecans, chopped or pieces (about 1 cup-------------------- 120 large halves).	118	3	810	11
527	Pumpkin and squash kernels, dry, 1 cup-------------------- hulled.	140	4	775	41
528	Sunflower seeds, dry, hulled------ 1 cup--------------------	145	5	810	35
	Walnuts:				
	Black:				
529	Chopped or broken kernels----- 1 cup--------------------	125	3	785	26
530	Ground (finely)--------------- 1 cup--------------------	80	3	500	16
531	Persian or English, chopped 1 cup-------------------- (about 60 halves).	120	4	780	18
	SUGARS AND SWEETS				
	Cake icings:				
	Boiled, white:				
532	Plain------------------------- 1 cup--------------------	94	18	295	1
533	With coconut------------------ 1 cup--------------------	166	15	605	3

Fat	Saturated (total)	Unsaturated		Carbohydrate	Calcium	Phosphorus	Iron	Potassium	Vitamin A value	Thiamin	Riboflavin	Niacin	Ascorbic acid
		Oleic	Linoleic										
(F)	(G)	(H)	(I)	(J)	(K)	(L)	(M)	(N)	(O)	(P)	(Q)	(R)	(S)
Grams	Grams	Grams	Grams	Grams	Milligrams	Milligrams	Milligrams	Milligrams	International units	Milligrams	Milligrams	Milligrams	Milligrams
1	0.2	0.1	0.5	88	18	100	3.3	109	0	0.74	0.46	6.1	0
1	.2	.1	.5	95	20	109	3.6	119	0	.80	.50	6.6	0
1	.1	.1	.3	76	16	70	2.8	91	0	.61	.38	5.1	0
1	.2	.1	.5	93	331	583	3.6	—	0	.80	.50	6.6	0
2	.4	.2	1.0	85	49	446	4.0	444	0	.66	.14	5.2	0
70	5.6	47.7	12.8	25	304	655	6.1	1,005	0	.31	1.20	4.6	Trace
62	5.0	42.2	11.3	22	269	580	5.4	889	0	.28	1.06	4.0	Trace
1	—	—	—	38	90	266	4.9	749	0	.25	.13	1.3	0
1	—	—	—	40	95	281	5.1	790	0	.27	.13	1.3	0
18	—	—	—	32	94	303	4.8	668	330	.18	.15	3.3	Trace
7	2.4	2.8	.6	48	138	235	4.6	536	330	.20	.08	1.5	5
12	4.3	5.0	1.1	54	161	291	5.9	—	—	.15	.10	1.3	—
1	—	—	—	42	74	278	4.6	673	10	.13	.10	1.5	—
1	—	—	—	49	55	293	5.9	1,163	—	.25	.11	1.3	—
1	—	—	—	35	43	238	3.3	573	30	.40	.10	1.0	—
19	4.8	6.2	7.1	3	53	196	1.0	203	Trace	.27	.03	.5	—
16	14.0	.9	.3	4	6	43	.8	115	0	.02	.01	.2	1
28	24.8	1.6	.5	8	10	76	1.4	205	0	.04	.02	.4	2
72	5.1	55.2	7.3	19	240	388	3.9	810	—	.53	—	1.0	Trace
Trace	—	—	—	39	50	238	4.2	498	40	.14	.12	1.2	0
72	13.7	33.0	20.7	27	107	577	3.0	971	—	.46	.19	24.8	0
8	1.5	3.7	2.3	3	9	61	.3	100	—	.02	.02	2.4	0
1	—	—	—	42	22	178	3.4	592	80	.30	.18	1.8	—
84	7.2	50.5	20.0	17	86	341	2.8	712	150	1.01	.15	1.1	2
65	11.8	23.5	27.5	21	71	1,602	15.7	1,386	100	.34	.27	3.4	—
69	8.2	13.7	43.2	29	174	1,214	10.3	1,334	70	2.84	.33	7.8	—
74	6.3	13.3	45.7	19	Trace	713	7.5	575	380	.28	.14	.9	—
47	4.0	8.5	29.2	12	Trace	456	4.8	368	240	.18	.09	.6	—
77	8.4	11.8	42.2	19	119	456	3.7	540	40	.40	.16	1.1	2
0	0	0	0	75	2	2	Trace	17	0	Trace	0.03	Trace	0
13	11.0	.9	Trace	124	10	50	0.8	277	0	0.02	.07	0.3	0

NUTRITIVE VALUES OF THE EDIBLE PART OF FOODS - Continued

(Dashes (—) denote lack of reliable data for a constituent believed to be present in measurable amount)

Item No. (A)	Foods, approximate measures, units, and weight (edible part unless footnotes indicate otherwise) (B)		Water (C)	Food energy (D)	Pro-tein (E)
		Grams	Per-cent	Cal-ories	Grams

SUGARS AND SWEETS —Con.

Cake icings —Continued
  Uncooked:

534	Chocolate made with milk and butter.	1 cup--------------------	275	14	1,035	9
535	Creamy fudge from mix and water.	1 cup--------------------	245	15	830	7
536	White-------------------------	1 cup--------------------	319	11	1,200	2
	Candy:					
537	Caramels, plain or chocolate----	1 oz---------------------	28	8	115	1
	Chocolate:					
538	Milk, plain-----------------	1 oz---------------------	28	1	145	2
539	Semisweet, small pieces (60 per oz).	1 cup or 6-oz pkg--------	170	1	860	7
540	Chocolate-coated peanuts--------	1 oz---------------------	28	1	160	5
541	Fondant, uncoated (mints, candy corn, other).	1 oz---------------------	28	8	105	Trace
542	Fudge, chocolate, plain---------	1 oz---------------------	28	8	115	1
543	Gum drops----------------------	1 oz---------------------	28	12	100	Trace
544	Hard--------------------------	1 oz---------------------	28	1	110	0
545	Marshmallows-------------------	1 oz---------------------	28	17	90	1
	Chocolate-flavored beverage powders (about 4 heaping tsp per oz):					
546	With nonfat dry milk-----------	1 oz---------------------	28	2	100	5
547	Without milk-------------------	1 oz---------------------	28	1	100	1
548	Honey, strained or extracted------	1 tbsp-------------------	21	17	65	Trace
549	Jams and preserves---------------	1 tbsp-------------------	20	29	55	Trace
550		1 packet-----------------	14	29	40	Trace
551	Jellies--------------------------	1 tbsp-------------------	18	29	50	Trace
552		1 packet-----------------	14	29	40	Trace
	Sirups:					
	Chocolate-flavored sirup or topping:					
553	Thin type---------------------	1 fl oz or 2 tbsp--------	38	32	90	1
554	Fudge type--------------------	1 fl oz or 2 tbsp--------	38	25	125	2
	Molasses, cane:					
555	Light (first extraction)------	1 tbsp-------------------	20	24	50	—
556	Blackstrap (third extraction)-	1 tbsp-------------------	20	24	45	—
557	Sorghum------------------------	1 tbsp-------------------	21	23	55	—
558	Table blends, chiefly corn, light and dark.	1 tbsp-------------------	21	24	60	0
	Sugars:					
559	Brown, pressed down-------------	1 cup--------------------	220	2	820	0
	White:					
560	Granulated--------------------	1 cup--------------------	200	1	770	0
561		1 tbsp-------------------	12	1	45	0
562		1 packet-----------------	6	1	23	0
563	Powdered, sifted, spooned into cup.	1 cup--------------------	100	1	385	0

VEGETABLE AND VEGETABLE PRODUCTS

Asparagus, green:
  Cooked, drained:
    Cuts and tips, 1 1/2- to 2-in lengths:

564	From raw--------------------	1 cup--------------------	145	94	30	3
565	From frozen-----------------	1 cup--------------------	180	93	40	6
	Spears, 1/2-in diam. at base:					
566	From raw--------------------	4 spears-----------------	60	94	10	1
567	From frozen-----------------	4 spears-----------------	60	92	15	2
568	Canned, spears, 1/2-in diam. at base.	4 spears-----------------	80	93	15	2
	Beans:					
	Lima, immature seeds, frozen, cooked, drained:					
569	Thick-seeded types (Fordhooks)	1 cup--------------------	170	74	170	10
570	Thin-seeded types (baby limas)	1 cup--------------------	180	69	210	13

		Fatty Acids												
			Unsaturated											
Fat	Satu-rated (total)	Oleic	Lino-leic	Carbo-hydrate	Calcium	Phos-phorus	Iron	Potas-sium	Vitamin A value	Thiamin	Ribo-flavin	Niacin	Ascorbic acid
(F)	(G)	(H)	(I)	(J)	(K)	(L)	(M)	(N)	(O)	(P)	(Q)	(R)	(S)
Grams	Grams	Grams	Grams	Grams	Milli-grams	Milli-grams	Milli-grams	Milli-grams	Inter-national units	Milli-grams	Milli-grams	Milli-grams	Milli-grams
38	23.4	11.7	1.0	185	165	305	3.3	536	580	.06	.28	.6	1
16	5.1	6.7	3.1	183	96	218	2.7	238	Trace	.05	.20	.7	Trace
21	12.7	5.1	.5	260	48	38	Trace	57	860	Trace	.06	Trace	Trace
3	1.6	1.1	.1	22	42	35	.4	54	Trace	.01	.05	.1	Trace
9	5.5	3.0	.3	16	65	65	.3	109	80	.02	.10	.1	Trace
61	36.2	19.8	1.7	97	51	255	4.4	553	30	.02	.14	.9	0
12	4.0	4.7	2.1	11	33	84	.4	143	Trace	.10	.05	2.1	Trace
1	.1	.3	.1	25	4	2	.3	1	0	Trace	Trace	Trace	0
3	1.3	1.4	.6	21	22	24	.3	42	Trace	.01	.03	.1	Trace
Trace	—	—	—	25	2	Trace	.1	1	0	0	Trace	Trace	0
Trace	—	—	—	28	6	2	.5	1	0	0	0	0	0
Trace	—	—	—	23	5	2	.5	2	0	0	Trace	Trace	0
1	.5	.3	Trace	20	167	155	.5	227	10	.04	.21	.2	1
1	.4	.2	Trace	25	9	48	.6	142	—	.01	.03	.1	0
0	0	0	0	17	1	1	.1	11	0	Trace	.01	.1	Trace
Trace	—	—	—	14	4	2	.2	18	Trace	Trace	.01	Trace	Trace
Trace	—	—	—	10	3	1	.1	12	Trace	Trace	Trace	Trace	Trace
Trace	—	—	—	13	4	1	.3	14	Trace	Trace	.01	Trace	1
Trace	—	—	—	10	3	1	.2	11	Trace	Trace	Trace	Trace	1
1	.5	.3	Trace	24	6	35	.6	106	Trace	.01	.03	.2	0
5	3.1	1.6	.1	20	48	60	.5	107	60	.02	.08	.2	Trace
—	—	—	—	13	33	9	.9	183	—	.01	.01	Trace	—
—	—	—	—	11	137	17	3.2	585	—	.02	.04	.4	—
—	—	—	—	14	35	5	2.6	—	—	—	.02	Trace	—
0	0	0	0	15	9	3	.8	1	0	0	0	0	0
0	0	0	0	212	187	42	7.5	757	0	.02	.07	.4	0
0	0	0	0	199	0	0	.2	6	0	0	0	0	0
0	0	0	0	12	0	0	Trace	Trace	0	0	0	0	0
0	0	0	0	6	0	0	Trace	Trace	0	0	0	0	0
0	0	0	0	100	0	0	.1	3	0	0	0	0	0
Trace	—	—	—	5	30	73	0.9	265	1,310	0.23	0.26	2.0	38
Trace	—	—	—	6	40	115	2.2	396	1,530	.25	.23	1.8	41
Trace	—	—	—	2	13	30	.4	110	540	.10	.11	.8	16
Trace	—	—	—	2	13	40	.7	143	470	.10	.08	.7	16
Trace	—	—	—	3	15	42	1.5	133	640	.05	.08	.6	12
Trace	—	—	—	32	34	153	2.9	724	390	.12	.09	1.7	29
Trace	—	—	—	40	63	227	4.7	709	400	.16	.09	2.2	22

NUTRIENTS IN INDICATED QUANTITY

NUTRITIVE VALUES OF THE EDIBLE PART OF FOODS · Continued

(Dashes (—) denote lack of reliable data for a constituent believed to be present in measurable amount)

Item No. (A)	Foods, approximate measures, units, and weight (edible part unless footnotes indicate otherwise) (B)		Water (C)	Food energy (D)	Pro- tein (E)
		Grams	Per- cent	Cal- ories	Grams

VEGETABLE AND VEGETABLE PRODUCTS—Con.

	Beans—Continued
	Snap:
	  Green:
	    Cooked, drained:				

571	From raw (cuts and French style).	1 cup-------------------- 125	92	30	2
	From frozen:				
572	Cuts--------------------	1 cup-------------------- 135	92	35	2
573	French style------------	1 cup-------------------- 130	92	35	2
574	Canned, drained solids (cuts).	1 cup-------------------- 135	92	30	2
	Yellow or wax: Cooked, drained:				
575	From raw (cuts and French style).	1 cup-------------------- 125	93	30	2
576	From frozen (cuts)-------	1 cup-------------------- 135	92	35	2
577	Canned, drained solids (cuts).	1 cup-------------------- 135	92	30	2
	Beans, mature. See Beans, dry (items 509-515) and Blackeye peas, dry (item 516). Bean sprouts (mung):				
578	Raw----------------------------	1 cup-------------------- 105	89	35	4
579	Cooked, drained----------------	1 cup-------------------- 125	91	35	4
	Beets: Cooked, drained, peeled:				
580	Whole beets, 2-in diam.-------	2 beets------------------ 100	91	30	1
581	Diced or sliced---------------	1 cup-------------------- 170	91	55	2
	Canned, drained solids:				
582	Whole beets, small------------	1 cup-------------------- 160	89	60	2
583	Diced or sliced--------------	1 cup-------------------- 170	89	65	2
584	Beet greens, leaves and stems, cooked, drained.	1 cup-------------------- 145	94	25	2
	Blackeye peas, immature seeds, cooked and drained:				
585	From raw-----------------------	1 cup-------------------- 165	72	180	13
586	From frozen--------------------	1 cup-------------------- 170	66	220	15
	Broccoli, cooked, drained: From raw:				
587	Stalk, medium size------------	1 stalk------------------ 180	91	45	6
588	Stalks cut into 1/2-in pieces-	1 cup-------------------- 155	91	40	5
	From frozen:				
589	Stalk, 4 1/2 to 5 in long-----	1 stalk------------------ 30	91	10	1
590	Chopped----------------------	1 cup-------------------- 185	92	50	5
	Brussels sprouts, cooked, drained:				
591	From raw, 7-8 sprouts (1 1/4- to 1 1/2-in diam.).	1 cup-------------------- 155	88	55	7
592	From frozen--------------------	1 cup-------------------- 155	89	50	5

	Cabbage:
	  Common varieties:
	    Raw:				

593	Coarsely shredded or sliced-	1 cup-------------------- 70	92	15	1
594	Finely shredded or chopped--	1 cup-------------------- 90	92	20	1
595	Cooked, drained---------------	1 cup-------------------- 145	94	30	2
596	Red, raw, coarsely shredded or sliced.	1 cup-------------------- 70	90	20	1
597	Savoy, raw, coarsely shredded or sliced.	1 cup-------------------- 70	92	15	2
598	Cabbage, celery (also called pe-tsai or wongbok), raw, 1-in pieces.	1 cup-------------------- 75	95	10	1
599	Cabbage, white mustard (also called bokchoy or pakchoy), cooked, drained.	1 cup-------------------- 170	95	25	2

		NUTRIENTS IN INDICATED QUANTITY											
		Fatty Acids											
Fat	Satu-rated (total)	Unsaturated Oleic	Lino-leic	Carbo-hydrate	Calcium	Phos-phorus	Iron	Potas-sium	Vitamin A value	Thiamin	Ribo-flavin	Niacin	Ascorbic acid
(F)	(G)	(H)	(I)	(J)	(K)	(L)	(M)	(N)	(O)	(P)	(Q)	(R)	(S)
Grams	Grams	Grams	Grams	Grams	Milli-grams	Milli-grams	Milli-grams	Milli-grams	Inter-national units	Milli-grams	Milli-grams	Milli-grams	Milli-grams
Trace	—	—	—	7	63	46	.8	189	680	.09	.11	.6	15
Trace	—	—	—	8	54	43	.9	205	780	.09	.12	.5	7
Trace	—	—	—	8	49	39	1.2	177	690	.08	.10	.4	9
Trace	—	—	—	7	61	34	2.0	128	630	.04	.07	.4	5
Trace	—	—	—	6	63	46	.8	189	290	.09	.11	.6	16
Trace	—	—	—	8	47	42	.9	221	140	.09	.11	.5	8
Trace	—	—	—	7	61	34	2.0	128	140	.04	.07	.4	7
Trace	—	—	—	7	20	67	1.4	234	20	.14	.14	.8	20
Trace	—	—	—	7	21	60	1.1	195	30	.11	.13	.9	8
Trace	—	—	—	7	14	23	.5	208	20	.03	.04	.3	6
Trace	—	—	—	12	24	39	.9	354	30	.05	.07	.5	10
Trace	—	—	—	14	30	29	1.1	267	30	.02	.05	.2	5
Trace	—	—	—	15	32	31	1.2	284	30	.02	.05	.2	5
Trace	—	—	—	5	144	36	2.8	481	7,400	.10	.22	.4	22
1	—	—	—	30	40	241	3.5	625	580	.50	.18	2.3	28
1	—	—	—	40	43	286	4.8	573	290	.68	.19	2.4	15
1	—	—	—	8	158	112	1.4	481	4,500	.16	.36	1.4	162
Trace	—	—	—	7	136	96	1.2	414	3,880	.14	.31	1.2	140
Trace	—	—	—	1	12	17	.2	66	570	.02	.03	.2	22
1	—	—	—	9	100	104	1.3	392	4,810	.11	.22	.9	105
1	—	—	—	10	50	112	1.7	423	810	.12	.22	1.2	135
Trace	—	—	—	10	33	95	1.2	457	880	.12	.16	.9	126
Trace	—	—	—	4	34	20	0.3	163	90	0.04	0.04	0.2	33
Trace	—	—	—	5	44	26	.4	210	120	.05	.05	.3	42
Trace	—	—	—	6	64	29	.4	236	190	.06	.06	.4	48
Trace	—	—	—	5	29	25	.6	188	30	.06	.04	.3	43
Trace	—	—	—	3	47	38	.6	188	140	.04	.06	.2	39
Trace	—	—	—	2	32	30	.5	190	110	.04	.03	.5	19
Trace	—	—	—	4	252	56	1.0	364	5,270	.07	.14	1.2	26

NUTRITIVE VALUES OF THE EDIBLE PART OF FOODS · Continued

(Dashes (—) denote lack of reliable data for a constituent believed to be present in measurable amount)

Item No. (A)	Foods, approximate measures, units, and weight (edible part unless footnotes indicate otherwise) (B)		Water (C)	Food energy (D)	Pro- tein (E)
		Grams	Per- cent	Cal- ories	Grams
	VEGETABLE AND VEGETABLE PRODUCTS—Con.				
	Carrots:				
	Raw, without crowns and tips, scraped:				
600	Whole, 7 1/2 by 1 1/8 in, or strips, 2 1/2 to 3 in long.	1 carrot or 18 strips---	72	88	30	1
601	Grated------------------------	1 cup--------------------	110	88	45	1
602	Cooked (crosswise cuts), drained	1 cup--------------------	155	91	50	1
	Canned:				
603	Sliced, drained solids--------	1 cup--------------------	155	91	45	1
604	Strained or junior (baby food)	1 oz (1 3/4 to 2 tbsp)--	28	92	10	Trace
	Cauliflower:				
605	Raw, chopped--------------------	1 cup--------------------	115	91	31	3
	Cooked, drained:				
606	From raw (flower buds)--------	1 cup--------------------	125	93	30	3
607	From frozen (flowerets)-------	1 cup--------------------	180	94	30	3
	Celery, Pascal type, raw:				
608	Stalk, large outer, 8 by 1 1/2 in, at root end.	1 stalk-----------------	40	94	5	Trace
609	Pieces, diced------------------	1 cup--------------------	120	94	20	1
	Collards, cooked, drained:				
610	From raw (leaves without stems)-	1 cup--------------------	190	90	65	7
611	From frozen (chopped)-----------	1 cup--------------------	170	90	50	5
	Corn, sweet:				
	Cooked, drained:				
612	From raw, ear 5 by 1 3/4 in---	1 ear[61]--------------	140	74	70	2
	From frozen:				
613	Ear, 5 in long-------------	1 ear[61]--------------	229	73	120	4
614	Kernels--------------------	1 cup--------------------	165	77	130	5
	Canned:				
615	Cream style--------------------	1 cup--------------------	256	76	210	5
	Whole kernel:				
616	Vacuum pack----------------	1 cup--------------------	210	76	175	5
617	Wet pack, drained solids----	1 cup--------------------	165	76	140	4
	Cowpeas. See Blackeye peas. (Items 585-586).				
	Cucumber slices, 1/8 in thick (large, 2 1/8-in diam.; small, 1 3/4-in diam.):				
618	With peel----------------------	6 large or 8 small slices	28	95	5	Trace
619	Without peel--------------------	6 1/2 large or 9 small pieces.	28	96	5	Trace
620	Dandelion greens, cooked, drained-	1 cup--------------------	105	90	35	2
621	Endive, curly (including escarole), raw, small pieces.	1 cup--------------------	50	93	10	1
	Kale, cooked, drained:				
622	From raw (leaves without stems and midribs).	1 cup--------------------	110	88	45	5
623	From frozen (leaf style)--------	1 cup--------------------	130	91	40	4
	Lettuce, raw:				
	Butterhead, as Boston types:				
624	Head, 5-in diam---------------	1 head[63]-------------	220	95	25	2
625	Leaves------------------------	1 outer or 2 inner or 3 heart leaves.	15	95	Trace	Trace
	Crisphead, as Iceberg:				
626	Head, 6-in diam---------------	1 head[64]-------------	567	96	70	5
627	Wedge, 1/4 of head-----------	1 wedge-----------------	135	96	20	1
628	Pieces, chopped or shredded---	1 cup--------------------	55	96	5	Trace
629	Looseleaf (bunching varieties including romaine or cos), chopped or shredded pieces.	1 cup--------------------	55	94	10	1
630	Mushrooms, raw, sliced or chopped-	1 cup--------------------	70	90	20	2
631	Mustard greens, without stems and midribs, cooked, drained.	1 cup--------------------	140	93	30	3
632	Okra pods, 3 by 5/8 in, cooked----	10 pods-----------------	106	91	30	2

[61]Weight includes cob. Without cob, weight is 77 g for item 612, 126 g for item 613.
[62]Based on yellow varieties. For white varieties, value is trace.
[63]Weight includes refuse of outer leaves and core. Without these parts, weight is 163 g.
[64]Weight includes core. Without core, weight is 539 g.

Fat (F)	Saturated (total) (G)	Unsaturated Oleic (H)	Unsaturated Linoleic (I)	Carbohydrate (J)	Calcium (K)	Phosphorus (L)	Iron (M)	Potassium (N)	Vitamin A value (O)	Thiamin (P)	Riboflavin (Q)	Niacin (R)	Ascorbic acid (S)
Grams	Grams	Grams	Grams	Grams	Milligrams	Milligrams	Milligrams	Milligrams	International units	Milligrams	Milligrams	Milligrams	Milligrams
Trace	—	—	—	7	27	26	.5	246	7,930	.04	.04	.4	6
Trace	—	—	—	11	41	40	.8	375	12,100	.07	.06	.7	9
Trace	—	—	—	11	51	48	.9	344	16,280	.08	.08	.8	9
Trace	—	—	—	10	47	34	1.1	186	23,250	.03	.05	.6	3
Trace	—	—	—	2	7	6	.1	51	3,690	.01	.01	.1	1
Trace	—	—	—	6	29	64	1.3	339	70	.13	.12	.8	90
Trace	—	—	—	5	26	53	.9	258	80	.11	.10	.8	69
Trace	—	—	—	6	31	68	.9	373	50	.07	.09	.7	74
Trace	—	—	—	2	16	11	.1	136	110	.01	.01	.1	4
Trace	—	—	—	5	47	34	.4	409	320	.04	.04	.4	11
1	—	—	—	10	357	99	1.5	498	14,820	.21	.38	2.3	144
1	—	—	—	10	299	87	1.7	401	11,560	.10	.24	1.0	56
1	—	—	—	16	2	69	.5	151	[62]310	.09	.08	1.1	7
1	—	—	—	27	4	121	1.0	291	[62]440	.18	.10	2.1	9
1	—	—	—	31	5	120	1.3	304	[62]580	.15	.10	2.5	8
2	—	—	—	51	8	143	1.5	248	[62]840	.08	.13	2.6	13
1	—	—	—	43	6	153	1.1	204	[62]740	.06	.13	2.3	11
1	—	—	—	33	8	81	.8	160	[62]580	.05	.08	1.5	7
Trace	—	—	—	1	7	8	.3	45	70	.01	.01	.1	3
Trace	—	—	—	1	5	5	0.1	45	Trace	0.01	0.01	0.1	3
1	—	—	—	7	147	44	1.9	244	12,290	.14	.17	—	19
Trace	—	—	—	2	41	27	.9	147	1,650	.04	.07	.3	5
1	—	—	—	7	206	64	1.8	243	9,130	.11	.20	1.8	102
1	—	—	—	7	157	62	1.3	251	10,660	.08	.20	.9	49
Trace	—	—	—	4	57	42	3.3	430	1,580	.10	.10	.5	13
Trace	—	—	—	Trace	5	4	.3	40	150	.01	.01	Trace	1
1	—	—	—	16	108	118	2.7	943	1,780	.32	.32	1.6	32
Trace	—	—	—	4	27	30	.7	236	450	.08	.08	.4	8
Trace	--	—	—	2	11	12	.3	96	180	.03	.03	.2	3
Trace	—	—	—	2	37	14	.8	145	1.050	.03	.04	.2	10
Trace	—	—	—	3	4	81	.6	290	Trace	.07	.32	2.9	2
1	—	—	—	6	193	45	2.5	308	8,120	.11	.20	.8	67
Trace	—	—	—	6	98	43	.5	184	520	.14	.19	1.0	21

NUTRIENTS IN INDICATED QUANTITY

NUTRITIVE VALUES OF THE EDIBLE PART OF FOODS · Continued

(Dashes (—) denote lack of reliable data for a constituent believed to be present in measurable amount)

Item No. (A)	Foods, approximate measures, units, and weight (edible part unless footnotes indicate otherwise) (B)		Water (C)	Food energy (D)	Protein (E)
			Percent	Calories	Grams
	VEGETABLE AND VEGETABLE PRODUCTS—Con.	Grams			
	Onions: Mature: Raw:				
633	Chopped	1 cup — 170	89	65	3
634	Sliced	1 cup — 115	89	45	2
635	Cooked (whole or sliced), drained.	1 cup — 210	92	60	3
636	Young green, bulb (3/8 in diam.) and white portion of top.	6 onions — 30	88	15	Trace
637	Parsley, raw, chopped	1 tbsp — 4	85	Trace	Trace
638	Parsnips, cooked (diced or 2-in lengths).	1 cup — 155	82	100	2
	Peas, green: Canned:				
639	Whole, drained solids	1 cup — 170	77	150	8
640	Strained (baby food)	1 oz (1 3/4 to 2 tbsp) — 28	86	15	1
641	Frozen, cooked, drained	1 cup — 160	82	110	8
642	Peppers, hot, red, without seeds, dried (ground chili powder, added seasonings).	1 tsp — 2	9	5	Trace
	Peppers, sweet (about 5 per lb, whole), stem and seeds removed:				
643	Raw	1 pod — 74	93	15	1
644	Cooked, boiled, drained	1 pod — 73	95	15	1
	Potatoes, cooked:				
645	Baked, peeled after baking (about 2 per lb, raw).	1 potato — 156	75	145	4
	Boiled (about 3 per lb, raw):				
646	Peeled after boiling	1 potato — 137	80	105	3
647	Peeled before boiling	1 potato — 135	83	90	3
	French-fried, strip, 2 to 3 1/2 in long:				
648	Prepared from raw	10 strips — 50	45	135	2
649	Frozen, oven heated	10 strips — 50	53	110	2
650	Hashed brown, prepared from frozen.	1 cup — 155	56	345	3
	Mashed, prepared from— Raw:				
651	Milk added	1 cup — 210	83	135	4
652	Milk and butter added	1 cup — 210	80	195	4
653	Dehydrated flakes (without milk), water, milk, butter, and salt added.	1 cup — 210	79	195	4
654	Potato chips, 1 3/4 by 2 1/2 in oval cross section.	10 chips — 20	2	115	1
655	Potato salad, made with cooked salad dressing.	1 cup — 250	76	250	7
656	Pumpkin, canned	1 cup — 245	90	80	2
657	Radishes, raw (prepackaged) stem ends, rootlets cut off.	4 radishes — 18	95	5	Trace
658	Sauerkraut, canned, solids and liquid.	1 cup — 235	93	40	2
	Southern peas. See Blackeye peas (items 585-586).				
	Spinach:				
659	Raw, chopped	1 cup — 55	91	15	2
	Cooked, drained:				
660	From raw	1 cup — 180	92	40	5
	From frozen:				
661	Chopped	1 cup — 205	92	45	6
662	Leaf	1 cup — 190	92	45	6
663	Canned, drained solids	1 cup — 205	91	50	6
	Squash, cooked:				
664	Summer (all varieties), diced, drained.	1 cup — 210	96	30	2

[65]Value based on white-fleshed varieties. For yellow-fleshed varieties, value in International Units (I.U.) is 70 for item 633, 50 for item 634, and 80 for item 635.

Fat	Fatty Acids			Carbo-hydrate	Calcium	Phos-phorus	Iron	Potas-sium	Vitamin A value	Thiamin	Ribo-flavin	Niacin	Ascorbic acid
	Satu-rated (total)	Unsaturated											
		Oleic	Lino-leic										
(F)	(G)	(H)	(I)	(J)	(K)	(L)	(M)	(N)	(O)	(P)	(Q)	(R)	(S)
Grams	Grams	Grams	Grams	Grams	Milli-grams	Milli-grams	Milli-grams	Milli-grams	Inter-national units	Milli-grams	Milli-grams	Milli-grams	Milli-grams
Trace	—	—	—	15	46	61	.9	267	[65]Trace	.05	.07	.3	17
Trace	—	—	—	10	31	41	.6	181	[65]Trace	.03	.05	.2	12
Trace	—	—	—	14	50	61	.8	231	[65]Trace	.06	.06	.4	15
Trace	—	—	—	3	12	12	.2	69	Trace	.02	.01	.1	8
Trace	—	—	—	Trace	7	2	.2	25	300	Trace	.01	Trace	6
1	—	—	—	23	70	96	.9	587	50	.11	.12	.2	16
1	—	—	—	29	44	129	3.2	163	1,170	.15	.10	1.4	14
Trace	—	—	—	3	3	18	.3	28	140	.02	.03	.3	3
Trace	—	—	—	19	30	138	3.0	216	960	.43	.14	2.7	21
Trace	—	—	—	1	5	4	.3	20	1,300	Trace	.02	.2	Trace
Trace	—	—	—	4	7	16	.5	157	310	.06	.06	.4	94
Trace	—	—	—	3	7	12	.4	109	310	.05	.05	.4	70
Trace	—	—	—	33	14	101	1.1	782	Trace	.15	.07	2.7	31
Trace	—	—	—	23	10	72	.8	556	Trace	.12	.05	2.0	22
Trace	—	—	—	20	8	57	.7	385	Trace	.12	.05	1.6	22
7	1.7	1.2	3.3	18	8	56	.7	427	Trace	.07	.04	1.6	11
4	1.1	.8	2.1	17	5	43	.9	326	Trace	.07	.01	1.3	11
18	4.6	3.2	9.0	45	28	78	1.9	439	Trace	.11	.03	1.6	12
2	.7	.4	Trace	27	50	103	8	548	40	.17	.11	2.1	21
9	5 6	2.3	0.2	26	50	101	0.8	525	360	0.17	0.11	2.1	19
7	3.6	2.1	.2	30	65	99	.6	601	270	.08	.08	1.9	11
8	2.1	1.4	4.0	10	8	28	.4	226	Trace	.04	.01	1.0	3
7	2.0	2.7	1.3	41	80	160	1.5	798	350	.20	.18	2.8	28
1	—	—	—	19	61	64	1.0	588	15,680	.07	.12	1.5	12
Trace	—	—	—	1	5	6	.2	58	Trace	.01	.01	.1	5
Trace	—	—	—	9	85	42	1.2	329	120	.07	.09	.5	33
Trace	—	—	—	2	51	28	1.7	259	4,460	.06	.11	.3	28
1	—	—	—	6	167	68	4.0	583	14,580	.13	.25	.9	50
1	—	—	—	8	232	90	4.3	683	16,200	.14	.31	.8	39
1	—	—	—	7	200	84	4.8	688	15,390	.15	.27	1.0	53
1	—	—	—	7	242	53	5.3	513	16,400	.04	.25	.6	29
Trace	—	—	—	7	53	53	.8	296	820	.11	.17	1.7	21

NUTRITIVE VALUES OF THE EDIBLE PART OF FOODS · Continued

(Dashes (—) denote lack of reliable data for a constituent believed to be present in measurable amount)

Item No. (A)	Foods, approximate measures, units, and weight (edible part unless footnotes indicate otherwise) (B)		Water (C)	Food energy (D)	Pro-tein (E)
			Grams	Per-cent	Cal-ories	Grams

VEGETABLE AND VEGETABLE PRODUCTS—Con.

			Grams	Percent	Calories	Grams
	Squash, cooked—Continued					
665	Winter (all varieties), baked, mashed.	1 cup--------------------	205	81	130	4
	Sweetpotatoes:					
	Cooked (raw, 5 by 2 in; about 2 1/2 per lb):					
666	Baked in skin, peeled---------	1 potato------------------	114	64	160	2
667	Boiled in skin, peeled--------	1 potato------------------	151	71	170	3
668	Candied, 2 1/2 by 2-in piece----	1 piece-------------------	105	60	175	1
	Canned:					
669	Solid pack (mashed)-----------	1 cup---------------------	255	72	275	5
670	Vacuum pack, piece 2 3/4 by 1 in.	1 piece-------------------	40	72	45	1
	Tomatoes:					
671	Raw, 2 3/5-in diam. (3 per 12 oz pkg.).	1 tomato⁶⁶---------------	135	94	25	1
672	Canned, solids and liquid-------	1 cup---------------------	241	94	50	2
673	Tomato catsup---------------------	1 cup---------------------	273	69	290	5
674		1 tbsp-------------------	15	69	15	Trace
	Tomato juice, canned:					
675	Cup-----------------------------	1 cup---------------------	243	94	45	2
676	Glass (6 fl oz)-----------------	1 glass-------------------	182	94	35	2
677	Turnips, cooked, diced-----------	1 cup---------------------	155	94	35	1
	Turnip greens, cooked, drained:					
678	From raw (leaves and stems)-----	1 cup---------------------	145	94	30	3
679	From frozen (chopped)-----------	1 cup---------------------	165	93	40	4
680	Vegetables, mixed, frozen, cooked-	1 cup---------------------	182	83	115	6

MISCELLANEOUS ITEMS

			Grams	Percent	Calories	Grams
	Baking powders for home use:					
	Sodium aluminum sulfate:					
681	With monocalcium phosphate monohydrate.	1 tsp--------------------	3.0	2	5	Trace
682	With monocalcium phosphate monohydrate, calcium sulfate.	1 tsp--------------------	2.9	1	5	Trace
683	Straight phosphate--------------	1 tsp--------------------	3.8	2	5	Trace
684	Low sodium----------------------	1 tsp--------------------	4.3	2	5	Trace
685	Barbecue sauce-------------------	1 cup--------------------	250	81	230	4
	Beverages, alcoholic:					
686	Beer-----------------------------	12 fl oz-----------------	360	92	150	1
	Gin, rum, vodka, whisky:					
687	80-proof-----------------------	1 1/2-fl oz jigger-------	42	67	95	—
688	86-proof-----------------------	1 1/2-fl oz jigger-------	42	64	105	—
689	90-proof-----------------------	1 1/2-fl oz jigger-------	42	62	110	—
	Wines:					
690	Dessert-------------------------	3 1/2-fl oz glass--------	103	77	140	Trace
691	Table---------------------------	3 1/2-fl oz glass--------	102	86	85	Trace
	Beverages, carbonated, sweetened, nonalcoholic:					
692	Carbonated water----------------	12 fl oz-----------------	366	92	115	0
693	Cola type-----------------------	12 fl oz-----------------	369	90	145	0
694	Fruit-flavored sodas and Tom Collins mixer.	12 fl oz-----------------	372	88	170	0
695	Ginger ale----------------------	12 fl oz-----------------	366	92	115	0
696	Root beer------------------------	12 fl oz-----------------	370	90	150	0
	Chili powder. See Peppers, hot, red (item 642).					

⁶⁶Weight includes cores and stem ends. Without these parts, weight is 123 g.
⁶⁷Based on year-round average. For tomatoes marketed from November through May, value is about 12 mg; from June through October, 32 mg.
⁶⁸Applies to product without calcium salts added. Value for products with calcium salts added may be as much as 63 mg for whole tomatoes, 241 mg for cut forms.

Fat	Fatty Acids			Carbo-hydrate	Calcium	Phos-phorus	Iron	Potas-sium	Vitamin A value	Thiamin	Ribo-flavin	Niacin	Ascorbic acid
	Satu-rated (total)	Unsaturated											
		Oleic	Lino-leic										
(F)	(G)	(H)	(I)	(J)	(K)	(L)	(M)	(N)	(O)	(P)	(Q)	(R)	(S)
Grams	Grams	Grams	Grams	Grams	Milli-grams	Milli-grams	Milli-grams	Milli-grams	Inter-national units	Milli-grams	Milli-grams	Milli-grams	Milli-grams
1	—	—	—	32	57	98	1.6	945	8,610	.10	.27	1.4	27
1	—	—	—	37	46	66	1.0	342	9,230	.10	.08	.8	25
1	—	—	—	40	48	71	1.1	367	11,940	.14	.09	.9	26
3	2.0	.8	.1	36	39	45	.9	200	6,620	.06	.04	.4	11
1	—	—	—	63	64	105	2.0	510	19,890	.13	.10	1.5	36
Trace	—	—	—	10	10	16	.3	80	3,120	.02	.02	.2	6
Trace	—	—	—	6	16	33	.6	300	1,110	.07	.05	.9	[67]28
Trace	—	—	—	10	[68]14	46	1.2	523	2,170	.12	.07	1.7	41
1	—	—	—	69	60	137	2.2	991	3,820	.25	.19	4.4	41
Trace	—	—	—	4	3	8	.1	54	210	.01	.01	.2	2
Trace	—	—	—	10	17	44	2.2	552	1,940	.12	.07	1.9	39
Trace	—	—	—	8	13	33	1.6	413	1,460	.09	.05	1.5	29
Trace	—	—	—	8	54	37	.6	291	Trace	.06	.08	.5	34
Trace	—	—	—	5	252	49	1.5	—	8,270	.15	.33	.7	68
Trace	—	—	—	6	195	64	2.6	246	11,390	.08	.15	.7	31
1	—	—	—	24	46	115	2.4	348	9,010	.22	.13	2.0	15
Trace	0	0	0	1	58	87	—	5	0	0	0	0	0
Trace	0	0	0	1	183	45	—	—	0	0	0	0	0
Trace	0	0	0	1	239	359	—	6	0	0	0	0	0
Trace	0	0	0	2	207	314	—	471	0	0	0	0	0
17	2.2	4.3	10.0	20	53	50	2.0	435	900	.03	.03	.8	13
0	0	0	0	14	18	108	Trace	90	—	.01	.11	2.2	—
—	0	0	0	Trace	—	—	—	1	—	—	—	—	—
—	0	0	0	Trace	—	—	—	1	—	—	—	—	—
—	0	0	0	Trace	—	—	—	1	—	—	—	—	—
0	0	0	0	8	8	—	—	77	—	.01	.02	.2	—
0	0	0	0	4	9	10	.4	94	—	Trace	.01	.1	—
0	0	0	0	29	—	—	—	—	0	0	0	0	0
0	0	0	0	37	--	—	—	—	0	0	0	0	0
0	0	0	0	45	—	—	—	—	0	0	0	0	0
0	0	0	0	29	—	—	—	0	0	0	0	0	0
0	0	0	0	39	—	—	—	0	0	0	0	0	0

NUTRITIVE VALUES OF THE EDIBLE PART OF FOODS - Continued

(Dashes (—) denote lack of reliable data for a constituent believed to be present in measurable amount)

Item No. (A)	Foods, approximate measures, units, and weight (edible part unless footnotes indicate otherwise) (B)		Water (C)	Food energy (D)	Protein (E)
		Grams	Percent	Calories	Grams
	MISCELLANEOUS ITEMS—Con.				
	Chocolate:				
697	Bitter or baking----------------	1 oz----------------------	28	2	145	3
	Semisweet, see Candy, chocolate (item 539).				
698	Gelatin, dry----------------------	1,7-g envelope-----------	7	13	25	6
699	Gelatin dessert prepared with gelatin dessert powder and water.	1 cup--------------------	240	84	140	4
700	Mustard, prepared, yellow---------	1 tsp or individual serving pouch or cup.	5	80	5	Trace
	Olives, pickled, canned:				
701	Green-----------------------------	4 medium or 3 extra large or 2 giant.[69]	16	78	15	Trace
702	Ripe, Mission--------------------	3 small or 2 large[69]-----	10	73	15	Trace
	Pickles, cucumber:				
703	Dill, medium, whole, 3 3/4 in long, 1 1/4-in diam.	1 pickle-----------------	65	93	5	Trace
704	Fresh-pack, slices 1 1/2-in diam., 1/4 in thick.	2 slices-----------------	15	79	10	Trace
705	Sweet, gherkin, small, whole, about 2 1/2 in long, 3/4-in diam.	1 pickle-----------------	15	61	20	Trace
706	Relish, finely chopped, sweet---	1 tbsp--------------------	15	63	20	Trace
	Popcorn. See items 476-478.				
707	Popsicle, 3-fl oz size------------	1 popsicle---------------	95	80	70	0
	Soups:				
	Canned, condensed:				
	Prepared with equal volume of milk:				
708	Cream of chicken------------	1 cup--------------------	245	85	180	7
709	Cream of mushroom-----------	1 cup--------------------	245	83	215	7
710	Tomato----------------------	1 cup--------------------	250	84	175	7
	Prepared with equal volume of water:				
711	Bean with pork--------------	1 cup--------------------	250	84	170	8
712	Beef broth, bouillon, consomme.	1 cup--------------------	240	96	30	5
713	Beef noodle-----------------	1 cup--------------------	240	93	65	4
714	Clam chowder, Manhattan type (with tomatoes, without milk).	1 cup--------------------	245	92	80	2
715	Cream of chicken------------	1 cup--------------------	240	92	95	3
716	Cream of mushroom-----------	1 cup--------------------	240	90	135	2
717	Minestrone------------------	1 cup--------------------	245	90	105	5
718	Split pea-------------------	1 cup--------------------	245	85	145	9
719	Tomato----------------------	1 cup--------------------	245	91	90	2
720	Vegetable beef--------------	1 cup--------------------	245	92	80	5
721	Vegetarian------------------	1 cup--------------------	245	92	80	2
	Dehydrated:				
722	Bouillon cube, 1/2 in---------	1 cube-------------------	4	4	5	1
	Mixes:				
	Unprepared:				
723	Onion---------------------	1 1/2-oz pkg-------------	43	3	150	6
	Prepared with water:				
724	Chicken noodle------------	1 cup--------------------	240	95	55	2
725	Onion---------------------	1 cup--------------------	240	96	35	1
726	Tomato vegetable with noodles.	1 cup--------------------	240	93	65	1
727	Vinegar, cider--------------------	1 tbsp-------------------	15	94	Trace	Trace
728	White sauce, medium, with enriched flour.	1 cup--------------------	250	73	405	10
	Yeast:				
729	Baker's, dry, active------------	1 pkg--------------------	7	5	20	3
730	Brewer's, dry-------------------	1 tbsp-------------------	8	5	25	3

[69]Weight includes pits. Without pits, weight is 13 g for item 701, 9 g for item 702.
[70]Value may vary from 6 to 60 mg.

	Fatty Acids												
Fat	Satu-rated (total)	Unsaturated Oleic	Lino-leic	Carbo-hydrate	Calcium	Phos-phorus	Iron	Potas-sium	Vitamin A value	Thiamin	Ribo-flavin	Niacin	Ascorbic acid
(F)	(G)	(H)	(I)	(J)	(K)	(L)	(M)	(N)	(O)	(P)	(Q)	(R)	(S)
Grams	Grams	Grams	Grams	Grams	Milli-grams	Milli-grams	Milli-grams	Milli-grams	Inter-national units	Milli-grams	Milli-grams	Milli-grams	Milli-grams
15	8.9	4.9	.4	8	22	109	1.9	235	20	.01	.07	.4	0
Trace	0	0	0	0	—	—	—	—	—	—	—	—	—
0	0	0	0	34	—	—	—	—	—	—	—	—	—
Trace	—	—	—	Trace	4	4	.1	7	—	—	—	—	—
2	.2	1.2	.1	Trace	8	2	.2	7	40	—	—	—	—
2	.2	1.2	.1	Trace	9	1	.1	2	10	Trace	Trace	—	—
Trace	—	—	—	1	17	14	.7	130	70	Trace	.01	Trace	4
Trace	—	—	—	3	5	4	.3	—	20	Trace	Trace	Trace	1
Trace	—	—	—	5	2	2	.2	—	10	Trace	Trace	Trace	1
Trace	—	—	—	5	3	2	.1	—	—	—	—	—	—
0	0	0	0	18	0	—	Trace	—	0	0	0	0	0
10	4.2	3.6	1.3	15	172	152	0.5	260	610	0.05	0.27	0.7	2
14	5.4	2.9	4.6	16	191	169	.5	279	250	.05	.34	.7	1
7	3.4	1.7	1.0	23	168	155	.8	418	1,200	.10	.25	1.3	15
6	1.2	1.8	2.4	22	63	128	2.3	395	650	.13	.08	1.0	3
0	0	0	0	3	Trace	31	.5	130	Trace	Trace	.02	1.2	—
3	.6	.7	.8	7	7	48	1.0	77	50	.05	.07	1.0	Trace
3	.5	.4	1.3	12	34	47	1.0	184	880	.02	.02	1.0	—
6	1.6	2.3	1.1	8	24	34	.5	79	410	.02	.05	.5	Trace
10	2.6	1.7	4.5	10	41	50	.5	98	70	.02	.12	.7	Trace
3	.7	.9	1.3	14	37	59	1.0	314	2,350	.07	.05	1.0	—
3	1.1	1.2	.4	21	29	149	1.5	270	440	.25	.15	1.5	1
3	.5	.5	1.0	16	15	34	.7	230	1,000	.05	.05	1.2	12
2	—	—	—	10	12	49	.7	162	2,700	.05	.05	1.0	—
2	—	—	—	13	20	39	1.0	172	2,940	.05	.05	1.0	—
Trace	—	—	—	Trace	—	—	—	4	—	—	—	—	—
5	1.1	2.3	1.0	23	42	49	.6	238	30	.05	.03	.3	6
1	—	—	—	8	7	19	.2	19	50	.07	.05	.5	Trace
1	—	—	—	6	10	12	.2	58	Trace	Trace	Trace	Trace	2
1	—	—	—	12	7	19	.2	29	480	.05	.02	.5	5
0	0	0	0	1	1	1	.1	15	—	—	—	—	—
31	19.3	7.8	.8	22	288	233	.5	348	1,150	.12	.43	.7	2
Trace	—	—	—	3	3	90	1.1	140	Trace	.16	.38	2.6	Trace
Trace	—	—	—	3	[70]17	140	1.4	152	Trace	1.25	.34	3.0	Trace

FOOD SOURCES OF ADDITIONAL NUTRIENTS

This chart shows the better food sources of some less common vitamins and minerals. Especially note the foods high in magnesium, a mineral that may be lacking in your diet if you eliminate milk.

This table is adapted from *Nutritive Value of Foods*, by Catherine F. Adams and Martha Richardson, prepared by the Science and Education Administration, United States Department of Agriculture, revised edition, April 1981.

FOOD SOURCES OF ADDITIONAL NUTRIENTS

VITAMINS

VITAMIN B$_6$	Vitamin B$_{12}$	Vitamin E
Bananas	(present in foods of animal origin only)	Vegetable oils
Whole-grain cereals		Margarine
Chicken	Kidney	Whole-grain cereals
Dry legumes	Liver	Peanuts
Most dark-green leafy vegetables	Meat	
	Milk	**Folacin**
Most fish and shellfish	Most cheese	Liver

278

Muscle meats, liver and kidney
Peanuts, walnuts, filberts, and peanut butter
Potatoes and sweetpotatoes
Prunes and raisins
Yeast

Most fish
Shellfish
Whole egg and egg yolk

Vitamin D

Vitamin D milks
Egg yolk
Saltwater fish
Liver

Dark-green vegetables
Dry beans
Peanuts
Wheat germ

MINERALS

Iodine

Iodized salt
Seafood

Magnesium

Bananas
Whole-grain cereals
Dry beans
Milk
Most dark-green vegetables
Nuts
Peanuts and peanut butter

Zinc

Shellfish
Meat
Poultry
Cheese
Whole-grain cereals
Dry beans
Cocoa
Nuts

INDEX

acidophilus milk, 82, 93, 116
acquired lactose intolerance, 150–51
  see also secondary lactose
    intolerance
alcoholic drinks, 190
alcoholism, 65, 172
allergy, *see* milk protein allergy
Americans, lactose intolerance in,
  17, 19, 21
Amerindians, lactose intolerance in,
  20–21, 28, 151
antacids, 168–69, 176
antibiotics, 54, 65
appetizers, 190
Arabs, lactose intolerance in, 21
arthritis, 171
Asians, lactose intolerance in,
  20–21, 151

babies:
  cramps in, 68
  development of intestines in, 148
  diarrhea in, 57, 67, 72, 153, 177
  glucose-galactose malabsorption
    in, 72–73, 153
  lactase production in, 147
  lactose intolerance in, 18, 57,
    146–53, 177
  milk protein allergy in, 65–71
  nutritional requirements of, 162–
    163, 171–72

baby food, 150
baby formulas, milk-free, 70, 103,
  155–58
Baskin-Robbins ice cream, 197
biopsy, 50–51
Blacks, lactose intolerance in, 19,
  21, 154
blood glucose test, 51–53
bone meal, 168
bread crumbs, 137, 192
breads and rolls, 134–35, 136–38,
  193
breakfast, 139, 199–200
breath test, *see* hydrogen breath test;
  carbon dioxide radioisotope
  breath test
butter, 84, 93, 116, 119
  substitutes for, *see* margarine
buttermilk, 82, 93, 116
  substitutes for, 98

caffeine, 135–36
cakes, 134, 138, 213–14
calcium, 167–71
  dietary requirements for, 20,
    32–33, 163, 173
  supplements for, 158, 168–69,
    174
calcium caseinate, 94, 96
Caltrate, 169
cancer, 62, 179

281